ALASKA'S
GALLEY WENCH
STYLE COOKING

RECIPES BY *ONY WOREL*
ARTWORK BY TINA MULCAHY CZT

Alaska's Galley Wench Style Cooking
Copyright © 2020 by Ony Worel

ISBN-13: 978-1-73495-500-2 (hardcover)

Credits
    Book Design: Workaday Communications
    Front Cover Photo: David Torreano
    Interior llustrations: Tina Mulcahy CZT
    Photo Editing: Lars Elling Lunde

I WOULD LIKE TO DEDICATE THIS BOOK TO:

My father, who gave me this beautiful way
of expressing my heart and my creativity;

My children, who are my whole world; and

Alaska's Kenai Peninsula, where I get to spend
the rest of my life falling in love with and
being inspired by its immeasurable beauty.

CONTENTS

DESSERTS

I spent my childhood training with my father, who was a great classically French-trained master chef. At the age of 14, I ran away to Alaska and it was love at first sight. From the moment I came to the Kenai, I was immersed in the beautiful, world-class, and quality local ingredients. I have dedicated myself to studying and adapting these ingredients with both traditional recipes and in my own inventions. For several years, my live radio show, The Galley Wench's Cooking Show, helped locals make use of what was fresh and in season. Some of the well-tested recipes from that show are in this very book -- along with other recipes I have worked at, practiced, and perfected with my family and friends.

This book is my best expression of how much I love and appreciate the Kenai Peninsula here in Alaska. My love of this beautiful place entwines with a love for cooking dishes with incredible ingredients that produce mind-blowing results. These are my best recipes, put together during my many years here. They are recipes made out of love and passion that taste cumtastic and have lots of character. They are recipes I hope will make you smile and inspired to cook with love like they do for me.

ONY WOREL

DRINKS & APPETIZERS

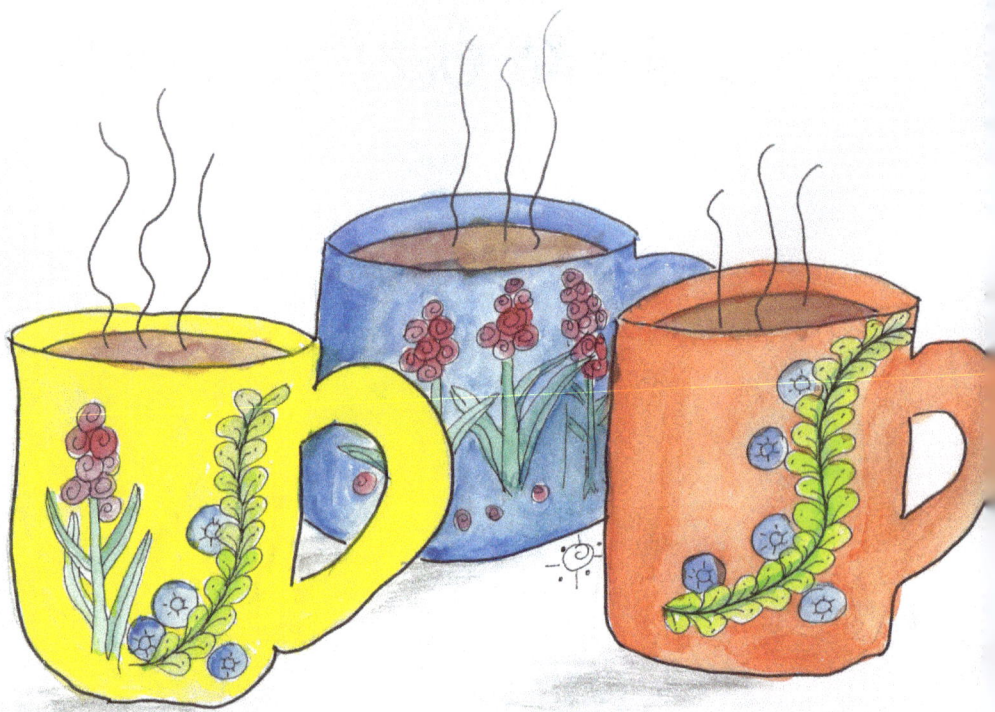

Wenches' Brew

INGREDIENTS:

- 6 oz. coconut juice
- 4 oz. guava juice
- 2 oz. pineapple juice
- 4 oz. 99 Bananas or other banana-flavor rum

DIRECTIONS:

Combine all ingredients and chill. Serve in coconut shell cups as is, on the rocks, or blended with a little umbrella and a straw.

Blushing Wench

INGREDIENTS:

- 2 oz. Malibu rum
- 2 oz. Chambord
- 4 oz. half & half, milk, or cream
- Ice

DIRECTIONS:

Combine all ingredients in a shaker, shake it up to chill, then pour over ice and serve. This drink is also pretty good blended.

The Galley Wench's Hot Butter Rum Batter for a Party

INGREDIENTS:

- 1 gal. real vanilla ice cream
- 1 lb. melted butter
- 2 c. packed dark-brown sugar
- 1 tbsp. cinnamon
- ½ tsp. nutmeg

DIRECTIONS:

In a large bowl with a hand mixer or in a stand mixer, whip the ice cream and brown sugar and the spices. Slowly add melted butter while it is still warm, and continue whipping until incorporated into the ice cream mixture completely. I usually store it in quart jars in the fridge.

The Galley Wench's Hot Butter Rum Batter Cocktail

INGREDIENTS:

- ¼ c. butter rum batter
- 2 oz. rum
- 4 oz. boiling water, tea, or coffee

DIRECTIONS:

Combine everything in a mug, stir well, and enjoy.

King Crab Pâté with Sauerkraut Cracker

INGREDIENTS:

- 2 lbs. crab meat
- 1 lb. unsalted butter
- ¼ c. finely chopped shallots
- 1 ½ tsp. beau monde
- 2 tbsp. dry vermouth
- 2 c. unbleached all-purpose flour
- 2 tbsp. unsalted butter
- 1 c. milk
- 1 c. sauerkraut drained and excess moisture squeezed out

DIRECTIONS:

TO MAKE PÂTÉ: Sauté shallots in the melted butter just until cooked, but be careful not to let the shallots caramelize. Add crab and beau monde to the butter, and heat just until hot. Transfer crab and butter to food processor, and process until smooth. Transfer to pâté dish or bowl, let cool to room temperature, and serve with sauerkraut crackers.

TO MAKE SAUERKRAUT CRACKERS:

In a food processor, add sauerkraut and process until very fine.

Add flour and butter and process until resembles fine meal. Add milk until it comes together as a dough ball that holds together.

Add additional milk by the tablespoon if needed. Divide dough into 3 pieces. On the back of an ungreased baking sheet, roll out a portion of the dough with plastic wrap on top of it until dough is very thin. It will look almost transparent. Carefully remove plastic wrap. With a knife cut dough, making squares. With a fork make wholes in each square. Bake in a preheated 325-degree oven for 20 to 25 minutes or until begins to turn golden brown. Remove to rack to cool, and repeat with the remaining dough. Serve with crab pâté.

CRAB PURSES WITH VANILLA SAUCE

INGREDIENTS:

- 1½ lbs. king crab meat
- 1 sheet puff pastry dough
  (thawed, cut in 6 equal squares, and rolled thin)
- 3 scallions sliced lengthwise
- 1 tbsp. butter
- 2 vanilla beans
- 1½ c. cream
- 2 tbsp. butter melted
- 3 egg yolks
- 2 tbsp. cane sugar
- salt & cayenne pepper

DIRECTIONS:

Sauté scallions until soft and let cool. Divide the king crab equally among the 6 squares of puff pastry, placing it in the center of pastry dough. Bring all 4 corners of the pastry to meet above the crab meat, and bunch them together so that you can tie them with a length of the sautéed scallion to make a little purse. Place each purse on a baking sheet, and bake in a 350-degree oven for 25 minutes or until puffed and golden brown. Remove from oven, and leave them on the baking sheet to make the sauce. In a double boiler, whisk the cream and eggs. Add the insides of the vanilla beans to the sauce by splitting them open and scraping out the insides with the back of a knife. As soon as the sauce begins to thicken, remove from the heat and whisk in the butter slowly. Season to taste with the salt & cayenne. Spoon sauce into the center of 6 serving dishes, and place a crab purse in the center of the sauce. Serves 6.

Soups & Stews

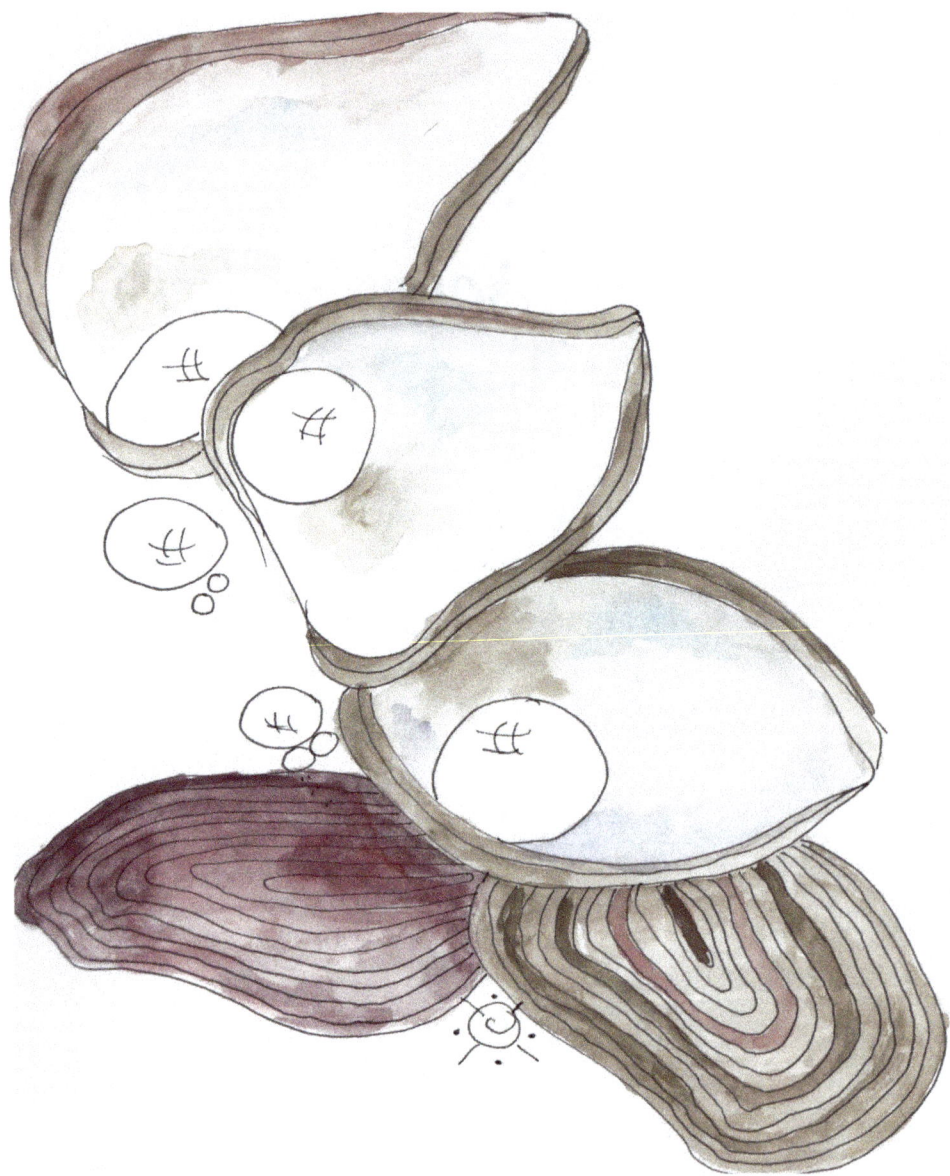

Oyster Stew

INGREDIENTS:

- 24 oysters, shucked, liquor reserved
- 3 tbsp. butter
- 2 tsp. finely diced shallots
- 1½ c. sliced oyster mushrooms
- ¼ c. dry vermouth
- 6 c. whole milk
- sea salt & fresh ground pepper

DIRECTIONS:

Sauté shallots in the butter in a soup pot. Add mushrooms and cook just till starts to soften. Add dry vermouth and bring to a boil. Add milk and bring just under a boil, then all at once add the oysters and reserved liquor, and heat back just under the boil. Taste and adjust seasoning with salt & pepper. Serve immediately in warm bowls. Serves 6 to 8.

Alaska King Crab Bisque

INGREDIENTS:

- 3 lbs. king crab meat medium diced
- 1 qt. half & half
- 1 qt. whole milk
- 4 tbsp. butter
- 4 tbsp. cornstarch
- kosher salt & cayenne pepper to taste

DIRECTIONS:

In a large double boiler, combine crab shells and the half & half. Steep the shells in the half & half and milk, occasionally stirring until hot. Turn off the heat, and let stand for 15 minutes. Strain and reserve hot milk mixture. Combine the melted butter and cornstarch to make a smooth paste in a pot, and cook over low heat for 2 minutes (do not allow to brown). Slowly add the hot milk to the butter and cornstarch while whisking. Continue stirring until thickened. Add the crab meat. Season with salt and cayenne pepper to taste, and serve hot or chill and serve cold. Serves 6 to 8.

Duck Barley Soup

INGREDIENTS:

- 1 roast duck
- ¼ c. duck fat
- 1 c. medium diced carrot
- 1 c. medium diced celery
- 1 c. medium diced leeks
- 1 c. medium diced sweet red pepper
- 2 c. medium diced mushrooms
- 4 unpeeled cloves of garlic
- 2 bay leaves
- 6 c. mushroom stock
- 1½ c. barley
- kosher salt & fresh ground black pepper

DIRECTIONS:

Remove the duck breasts from the duck with a sharp knife, and reserve for another preparation. Roast the rest of the duck for 1 hour at 375 degrees in oven. In a large soup pot add some of the duck fat from the roasted duck and all the vegetables, and cook on medium heat until they are sweated but not caramelized. Add roast duck to the pot and pour in the stock. Add the bay leaves and garlic cloves to the pot. Cook just under a simmer at a medium low to low heat for 1½ hours or until the duck meat falls off the bones and creates a beautiful broth. Carefully remove duck and garlic cloves from the soup pot, and set aside to cool. Add barley to the broth, raise the temperature to a boil, then reduce heat to a simmer once again. As soon as the duck is cool enough to handle, remove all the meat from the carcass, and return it to the soup pot. Also squeeze the garlic out of the peels, mash with a fork into a paste, and add it back to the soup. Cook another 35 to 45 minutes or until the barley is tender and the broth starts to thicken. You may need to add more broth if it gets too thick, so it doesn't scorch. Salt & pepper to taste.

Alaskan Wedding Soup

INGREDIENTS:

- 1 lb. ground moose meat
- 1 slice of white bread soaked with a little heavy cream
- 2 tbsp. cornstarch
- ¼ c. minced onion
- 1 tsp. minced or grated garlic
- ½ tsp. dried oregano
- ½ tsp. fresh finely chopped sage
- 1 large egg
- salt & pepper to taste
- 6 c. light stock
- 1 c. white wine
- 2 c. dried navy beans soaked and cooked tender
- 2 tbsp. olive oil
- 1 large onion, medium diced
- 2 large Alaskan carrots cut into rounds
- 2 c. dandelion greens or other greens like endive or kale, medium chopped, blanched tender
- bay leaf & sprig of fresh thyme

DIRECTIONS:

Combine the first 8 ingredients in a bowl for making little moose meatballs and reserve. In a large pot warm the olive oil. Add in the onions and carrots, and sweat until they just start to cook and change color. Pour in the stock, wine, bay leaf & thyme, and the beans. Bring to a gentle light boil. Taste for salt & pepper. Drop tiny moose meatballs from the meat mixture into the simmering stock. Make them ½ tsp. to 1 tsp. size. Simmer 5 minutes. Add greens and taste again for salt & pepper. Bring just to a boil, then turn it off and serve.

Braised Miso Halibut
with Toasted Rice Noodle

INGREDIENTS:

- 3 lbs. 2-inch halibut steaks cut into 6 pieces
- 9 c. clam juice or light stock
- ½ c. yellow miso paste
- ¼ c. sake
- ¼ c. fish sauce
- 2½ tbsp. garlic chili sauce
- ¼ c. sliced scallions
- 2 tbsp. peanut oil
- 2 tsp. fresh garlic, minced
- 2 tsp. fresh ginger, minced
- 1 lb. rice noodles
- toasted sesame seeds
- toasted walnut oil

DIRECTIONS:

In a soup pot warm the garlic and ginger in the peanut oil. Then add the stock, sake, fish sauce, and chili sauce to the soup pot, and bring it to a boil. Place noodles on a baking sheet, and toast in a 350-degree oven for 10 to 15 minutes or until starting to turn golden. Add noodles to boiling salted water, and cook just until tender. Strain noodles and divide into serving bowls. Reduce heat on the broth to a slow simmer. Rub the halibut with the miso to coat. In a hot nonstick pan add a little walnut oil, sear one side of the halibut in the skillet, then place it in a deep baking pan with the browned side up in one layer. Bring the broth to a rolling boil. Pour boiling broth into the pan with the fish but not over the fish, just halfway up the side of the pieces of fish. Let set for 6 to 8 minutes. Lay piece of halibut on top of noodles in the bowls. Heat broth back up just under a boil, and ladle over the fish. Garnish with the sliced scallions and toasted sesame seeds. Serves 6.

Moose Stew

INGREDIENTS:

- 2 lbs. moose meat cut in 2-inch cubes
- salt & pepper to taste
- ¼ c. gin
- peel of 1 orange
- 2 tbsp. rosemary
- 2 cloves garlic, bashed and peeled
- 1 c. flour
- ¼ lb. bacon
- ¼ c. bacon fat
- 1 can tomato paste
- 1 large red onion, large dice
- 4 medium carrots, large dice
- 2 bulbs fresh fennel, large dice
- 2 bell peppers, 1 gold, 1 red, large dice
- 1 lb. red, blue, or yellow fin (one or combination of all is nice), large dice
- 1 c. maple syrup
- 1 Alaskan Pale Ale or Pete's Wicked Ale
- 4 c. moose stock or beef stock
  (additional stock if needed during cooking)
- 3 bay leaves

DIRECTIONS:

Marinate the moose in the gin, orange peel, rosemary, salt & pepper, and garlic for 1 hour.

In a large pot (cast-iron Dutch oven is best), add the bacon and cook until it is slightly crisp but not hard, remove the bacon, leaving the bacon fat in the pot and adding additional bacon fat if needed, sear the meat in the bacon fat, then reserve it to a warm plate. Add the tomato paste to the drippings and sauté it, stirring constantly so it does not scorch but begins to brown. Stir in all the vegetables, syrup, ale, and stock. Add the bay leaves. Bring to a boil, and cook at a very low simmer for 1½ to 2 hours. Serve with fresh baked bread.

THE BEST MOOSE CHILI, ALASKA STYLE

INGREDIENTS:

- 4 fat dry high THC buds removed from stems and finely powdered in a coffee bean grinder
- 3 lbs. ground moose meat
- ¼ c. bacon drippings
- 4 c. pinto beans, cooked just tender but not mushy and drained
- 2 c. onions, medium diced
- 6 dried ancho peppers toasted, soaked in hot water until soft, then pureed into a paste
- 2 bay leaves
- ¼ cup cumin seeds, toasted, then freshly ground
- 1 bulb garlic, peeled, cloves quartered
- 1 or more fresh serrano peppers, toasted until skin is browned, left whole
- salt & fresh ground pepper to taste
- 3 c. moose bone broth or beef bone broth

DIRECTIONS:

In a big pot melt the bacon drippings, and get it hot. Add onions, and sauté until tender and all the water is cooked out and they start to brown. Add ancho paste, cumin, weed powder, garlic, and cumin. Continue stirring until the spices become fragrant. Add the moose meat to the onion and spices, and cook just until medium rare but not all the way through. Time to add the beans and the broth. Cook on a slow simmer for 45 minutes, stirring occasionally until the chili becomes thick, and serve. Leftovers freeze well for future use. It gets even better the next day.

(Optional: Can be made without the THC)

Fireweed Stew

INGREDIENTS:

- 2 c. fireweed shoots and tender tops
- 3 c. purple potatoes
- 8 slices of bacon, medium dice
- 1 c. celery
- 1 c. onion
- 1 c. finely diced chanterelle mushrooms, fresh or dried reconstituted
- bay leaf
- 6 c. light stock
- 1 pt. heavy cream
- ¼ c. cornstarch mixed with ⅔ c. dry vermouth
- 1 tbsp. raw sugar
- sea salt & fresh ground pepper to taste
- 2 tbsp. soft butter

DIRECTIONS:

In a big pot render the bacon at medium heat, and get it golden brown but not crispy. Add the celery and onion, and continue cooking until they start to cook and change color. Add potatoes, and stir frequently so the vegetables begin to cook but not caramelizing. Pour in stock, salt & pepper to taste, and put in the sugar. Simmer 20 minutes or just until the potatoes start to become tender. Once the potatoes are tender, add the heavy cream and vermouth with the cornstarch. Bring to a simmer for 2 to 5 minutes until thickened and starch taste is gone. Taste again for seasoning. Just before serving, stir in the butter.

GALLEY WENCH'S RECIPE
FOR TRADITIONAL CLAM CHOWDER

INGREDIENTS:

- 4 slices salt pork, small diced
- 1½ c. onion, medium small diced
- ¾ c. celery, medium small diced
- 1½ c. clam juice
- 4 c. cubed red skin potatoes
- 2 tsp. salt
- fresh ground black pepper to taste
- 2 c. whole milk
- 1 c. cold half & half
- 1 c. heavy cream
- 3 tbsp. butter
- 2 c. fresh clams or canned
- ½ c. dry vermouth

DIRECTIONS:

Sauté the salt pork on medium heat in a good-sized soup pot until lightly brown, add the onions and celery, reduce heat; sweat the vegetables, making sure not to let them brown, just until they are almost transparent. Add the potatoes and the clam juice, bring just to a simmer, cook 20 to 25 minutes or until the potatoes are just tender, add the clams, cook 3 to 5 minutes, add the milk, half & half, heavy cream, vermouth, and bring to a simmer for another 2 to 3 minutes. Remove from the heat. Stir in butter just before serving.

Main Courses & Side Dishes

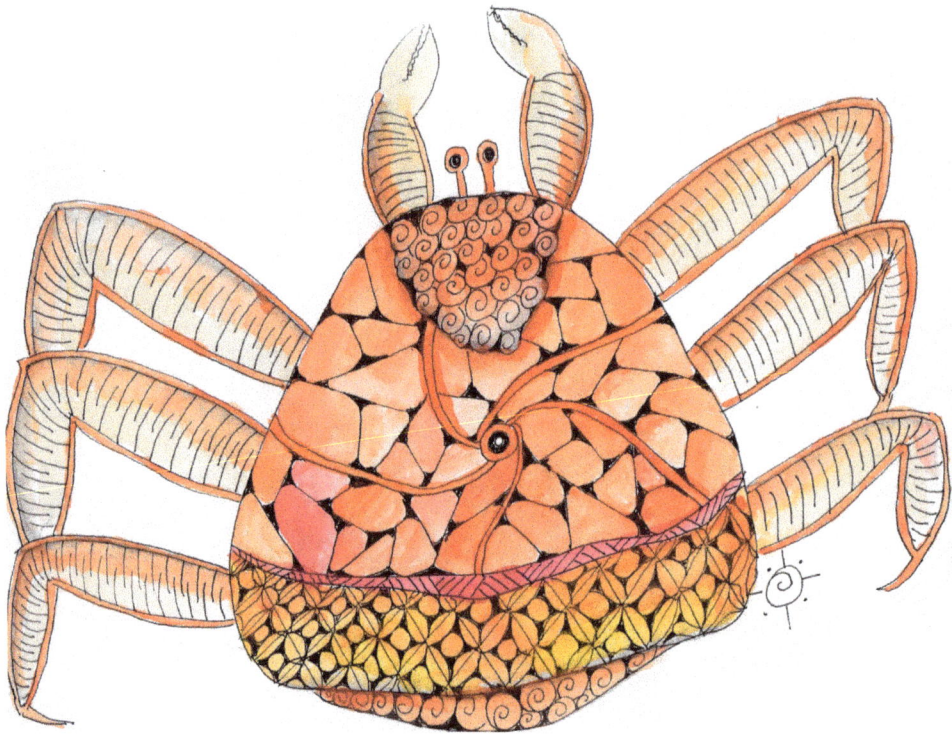

Smoked Salmon & Mascarpone Pie

INGREDIENTS:

- 1 lb. very thinly sliced smoked salmon
- 1 lb. mascarpone cheese, room temperature, and whipped with an electric mixer until fluffy
- 1 sheet frozen puff pastry, thawed, rolled, and cut in an 8-inch circle to fit in an 8-inch spring form pan
- 1 egg
- $\frac{1}{4}$ c. milk
- 1 small sweet red onion, diced fine
- 3 hardboiled eggs, diced fine
- $\frac{1}{4}$ c. finely chopped chives
- $\frac{1}{4}$ c. finely chopped capers
- wax paper

DIRECTIONS:

In the spring form pan, place the puff pastry. Prick the pastry with a fork. Beat the milk and egg to make an egg wash. Brush the egg wash on the puff pastry. Bake the pastry in a preheated 350-degree oven for 15 to 20 minutes or until golden brown. Remove pastry to wire rack to cool. Cut a piece of wax paper to fit around the ring of the spring form pan. Place the wax paper around the inside of the spring form pan against the ring with the shiny side in. Place cooled pastry back in spring form pan. Spread the mascarpone cheese over the pastry. From the center spiraling outward, layer the smoked salmon to cover the cheese. Make a border of the diced eggs around the outer edge of the salmon. Next, make another row around with the red onions leaving a little space to see the salmon beneath. Leaving another small space, go around with the chives. Finish off with the capers in the middle, making a circle. Cover lightly with plastic wrap, and refrigerate for 1 hour or until ready to serve. When ready to serve remove from spring form pan, and gently remove the wax paper. Slice in pie shape slices and serve.

Pork Loin Roasted on a Bed of Turnips & Apples
Finished with a Rosemary, Raisin Cream Sauce

INGREDIENTS:

- 4 lbs. pork loin roast
- 1/2 c. turbinado sugar
- 1/4 c. kosher salt
- 2 tbsp. freshly ground black pepper
- 4 to 5 medium-sized turnips, peeled, large diced
- 2 apples, peeled and cored, large diced
- 1 c. raisins
- 2 c. water
- 1/4 c. melted butter & 1/4 c. flour stirred together to make a paste
- 1 c. heavy cream
- 1 tsp. finely chopped fresh rosemary

DIRECTIONS:

In a bowl combine the sugar, salt, & black pepper to make a dry rub for the pork roast. Rub pork roast all over with the dry rub, and let sit in fridge for 1 hour or overnight. Put pork roast into Dutch oven or covered roaster. Surround the roast with the turnips & apples. Sprinkle in the raisins. Pour in the water, and roast in a 350-degree oven for 2 1/2 to 3 hours. Remove roast from pan to serving plate, and let rest at least 20 minutes before carving. Remove apples and turnips to a warm serving dish, and keep warm for the table. On stovetop on high heat, bring liquid in the Dutch oven to a boil, and reduce slightly. Using a whisk, add flour and butter paste, cooking until thick and bubbly, stirring constantly, and reduce heat if needed (needs to boil 2 minutes to get rid of starchy taste). Slowly stir in the cream and cook until hot. Before removing from heat, add the rosemary and give a last stir. Taste for seasoning. Pour sauce into a gravy boat or warm bowl, and serve with your roast.

CASHEW CRUSTED KODIAK SCALLOPS

INGREDIENTS:

- 24 fresh jumbo Kodiak scallops
- 1½ c. finely chopped cashews (unsalted)
- ¼ c. wasabi paste
- fresh ground black pepper & salt
- ¼ c. rose hip jelly
- 1½ c. heavy cream
- ¼ c. sunflower oil

DIRECTIONS:

Pat dry scallops with paper towels. Rub one side of the scallops with the wasabi. Sprinkle the wasabi side of the scallops lightly with salt & pepper, and then press the same side into the chopped cashews gently. Set aside. Heat sunflower oil to medium high heat, and sear the side without the cashews for about 2 to 3 minutes; reduce heat to low, turn over scallops, and cook another 2 to 3 minutes, being careful not to let the cashews get too dark. Remove to warm plate and make sauce. Warm the cream just until hot over medium-low heat. Transfer to a blender and add the rose hip jelly. Blend until smooth and foamy. Spoon onto the center of your plates, and arrange 3 scallops on top of the sauce and serve. Serves 6.

ROSE HIP JELLY

DIRECTIONS:

Pick only the red, plump, ripe hips. Gather a bagful of hips; wash and dry them. Cut them in halves, lengthwise. Put them into a preserving kettle with a small amount of water. Cover and cook until tender, watching to see that they do not burn. Add a little more water if necessary.

Strain through a jelly bag.

Measure the liquid and boil it for 10 minutes. Then add 1 pound of raw sugar to each pint of juice you have, and boil until it gels well when a spoonful is put on a plate. Then bottle and seal.

Swedish Moose Meatballs

INGREDIENTS:

- 2 lbs. ground moose burger
- 3 slices fresh white bread
- vermouth (enough to soak the bread)
- 1/4 c. butter
- 1/2 c. finely minced onion
- 1/4 c. grated carrot
- 6 cloves garlic minced
- 2 tbsp. cornstarch
- 1 egg
- 2 tsp. caraway seeds toasted
- salt & pepper to taste

FOR THE SAUCE:

- 1/4 c. flour
- 1/2 c. butter
- 2 c. moose or beef stock
- 1 c. sour cream or buttermilk

DIRECTIONS:

TO MAKE THE MEATBALLS: Sweat the onion, garlic, and carrot in the butter until tender and starting to caramelize. Combine the caramelized vegetables with the meat, egg, and caraway seeds. Form the meatballs, place on a plate, and refrigerate for 30 minutes to 1 hour to let meat absorb some of the flavors of the seasonings. Sauté the meatballs in a good enough amount of butter that you will have some left over to make your roux for the sauce. Set meatballs aside and make the sauce.

TO MAKE THE SAUCE: Add the flour to the butter left from browning the meatballs to make a roux. Cook, stirring the roux 2 minutes to cook out the starchy taste from the flour. Slowly add your stock, stirring constantly to prevent lumps. Continue adding liquid as the sauce thickens until it is the consistency of pancake batter. Add your sour cream or buttermilk while still stirring. As soon as the sauce starts to bubble, add back the meatballs, and put in a 350-degree oven, lightly covered with parchment paper. Bake for 20 to 25 minutes, testing a meatball before you turn off the oven to make sure it is cooked through. Serve with buttered egg noodles, rice, or mashed potatoes.

Moose Scallops in Buttermilk Béchamel Sauce

INGREDIENTS:

- 3 lbs. moose backstrap or tenderloin in 1/2-inch steaks, pounded flat
- 1/2 medium-sized red onion, sliced thin
- 1/2 red sweet bell pepper, sliced thin
- 1/2 green bell pepper, sliced thin
- 3 tbsp. butter
- olive oil
- flour
- kosher salt & white pepper
- béchamel sauce:
- 1/4 c. unsalted butter
- 1/4 c. all-purpose unbleached flour
- 1 1/2 c. scalded buttermilk
- 1/2 c. scalded cream
- 1 small onion studded with 2 cloves
- salt & nutmeg to taste

DIRECTIONS:

TO MAKE SAUCE: Combine buttermilk and cream in a saucepan, bring just under a boil on medium heat while stirring, and set aside. Melt butter until it just starts to foam, and add the flour, stirring until it is combined with the melted butter. Cook over medium-low heat for 2 minutes, making a light roux. Stir scalded buttermilk cream mixture slowly into the roux, and simmer until it starts to thicken. Add studded onion, and simmer about 20 minutes, keeping it stirred. Strain and reserve.

TO MAKE MOOSE SCALLOPS: Melt butter with the oil on medium heat. Season moose scallops with the salt & white pepper, and dredge them lightly in the flour. Sauté the moose until lightly golden brown. This will not take very long, and care needs to be taken so as not to have too hot of a pan that it will scorch the flour and make it bitter yet not cook the moose. Remove moose as it is browned to a warm plate. In the same pan, while it is still hot, add the peppers and onions. Cook until wilted but not caramelized. Add moose back to skillet, and pour over béchamel sauce. Simmer on medium low heat until bubbly, and serve.

MERLOT MARINATED PEPPER-CRUSTED TENDERLOIN
OF MOOSE ON A PLANK WITH ROASTED BABY VEGETABLES
& RHUBARB HORSERADISH RELISH

INGREDIENTS:

- 3½ to 4 lbs. moose tenderloin
- 2 c. merlot
- kosher salt
- 1 c. coarsely ground fresh black pepper
- 2 c. baby sweet peppers
- 2 c. baby carrots, blanched until tender crisp
- 2 c. peeled pearl onions, blanched until tender
- 2 c. new potatoes, blanched until tender
- ¼ c. sunflower oil
- 2 c. fresh rhubarb, small dice
- ¼ c. horseradish root, shredded fresh
- ½ c. fresh fennel, small dice
- ¼ c. red onion, small dice
- ¼ c. golden raisins
- ¼ c. raw cane sugar
- 2 tbsp. apple cider vinegar
- 1 tbsp. virgin olive oil

DIRECTIONS:

Marinate 4 to 6 hours or overnight the tenderloin in the merlot. Heat oven and plank to 350. Remove moose from the marinade and season liberally with the salt, then roll in the black pepper to cover entirely, pressing to embed the pepper into the meat. Sear over medium-high heat in a hot skillet all sides, and place on the center of preheated-to-375-degrees cedar plank. Toss the baby vegetables in the sunflower oil, season with salt & pepper to taste, place around the moose on the plank, and return to the 375-degree oven. Roast for 25 minutes, then turn off the oven.

Leave it in the oven undisturbed (do not open the door of the oven) for 30 minutes. Transfer the tenderloin to a plate to rest, and keep the vegetables warm in the oven. Slice moose meat, and toss the vegetables in a little butter. Return the sliced moose to plank with the vegetables, and serve with the relish in the following recipe. Serves 6.

TO MAKE RELISH: In a medium saucepan, combine rhubarb, onion, fennel, raisins, and olive oil. Sauté until tender, then add cane sugar, salt & pepper, and cider vinegar. Cook until liquid is reduced, remove from heat, let cool completely, and stir in horseradish root. Serve as a condiment with moose tenderloin or any game meat.

Pistachio Crusted Halibut
with Sweet Avocado Coulee

INGREDIENTS:

- 6 2-inch halibut steaks
- 1½ c. finely chopped pistachios
- 1½ c. sourdough breadcrumbs
- 2 cloves garlic, minced
- ¼ tsp. cayenne pepper
- ½ tsp. dry wasabi powder
- salt
- 1 c. unbleached all-purpose flour
- 2 eggs
- ½ c. milk
- ¼ c. clarified butter
- 2 avocados, pitted, peeled, and diced
- 1 c. heavy cream
- ¼ c. Alaska birch syrup
- 2 tsp. fresh lemon juice
- lime wedges

DIRECTIONS:

Butter a baking sheet with the clarified butter, and preheat oven to 400 degrees. Season each steak with salt, cayenne, and wasabi powder, and dredge one side of the steaks in flour. Combine breadcrumbs, pistachios, and garlic on a plate. Beat together eggs and milk in a pie plate. Dip the floured side of halibut steaks in the egg mixture, then press it into the pistachio mixture. Place with pistachio side up on baking sheet. Bake for 18 to 20 minutes or until halibut is cooked through and crust begins to brown. In a blender, blend the avocados, cream, and syrup. Add to the blender the lemon juice. Season with salt & cayenne pepper to taste. Spoon avocado sauce on serving plates, place halibut steak on top, garnish with lime wedges. Serves 6.

PANCETTA-WRAPPED KODIAK SCALLOPS
FINISHED WITH DRY SHERRY

INGREDIENTS:
- 24 Kodiak scallops
- kosher salt
- fresh ground black pepper
- 6 garlic cloves
- 12 slices pancetta, cut in half
- ½ c. dry sherry

DIRECTIONS:

In a small bowl combine the salt, pepper, and garlic. With the back of a fork, or if you have a mortar and pestle, use the salt & pepper against the garlic to mince it into a fine paste. Rub this mixture on your scallops. Wrap each scallop with a piece of the pancetta, and secure with a toothpick. Sauté the scallops at high heat until the pancetta is cooked. Remove scallops to a serving plate, deglaze the pan with the sherry, adding additional butter if desired, and pour over the scallops. Serves 6 for appetizer; double recipe for a meal.

The Galley Wench's Smoked Salmon

INGREDIENTS:

- 4 salmon fillets
- ¼ c. chopped garlic
- ¼ c. fresh sliced ginger
- 2 c. soy sauce
- 2 c. plum wine
- 1½ c. cane sugar or firmly packed brown sugar

DIRECTIONS:

Combine the garlic, ginger, soy sauce, wine, and sugar in a bowl, and stir until sugar is dissolved. Pour brine over salmon fillets in a glass dish, or you can use zipper bags, making sure they are closed tightly, and put them on a baking sheet in case of leaks. Marinate in the fridge overnight. Remove from the marinade, place on smoker racks, and let them sit until the fish dries off and becomes tacky. Smoke 6 to 8 hours in a cold smoker, 2 to 3 hours in a hot smoker.

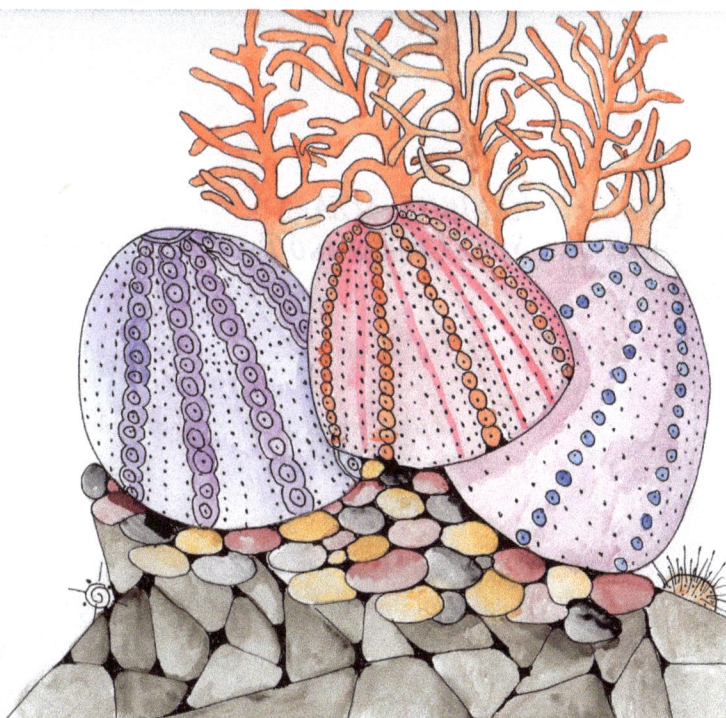

CHIPOTLE SMOKED SALMON
(DRY RUB METHOD RECIPE FOR SMOKED SALMON)

INGREDIENTS:

- 4 salmon fillets
- 1 c. kosher salt or the Galley Wench's Smoked Salt
- ¾ c. turbinado sugar
- 1 tbsp. Mexican oregano
- 1 tbsp. fresh chopped cilantro
- 2 tbsp. granulated garlic
- 2 tbsp. toasted ground cumin seeds
- ¼ c. ground dried ancho peppers
- ¼ c. ground chipotle peppers
- ¼ c. fresh ground toasted black pepper

DIRECTIONS:

Combine all dried ingredients in a bowl. Rub the salmon generously with the dry rub to coat it completely. Set the fillets in a glass dish or in zipper bags overnight in the refrigerator. Brush off excess rub from the salmon fillets, and place on smoker racks. Cold smoker for 6 to 8 hours, hot smoker for 2 to 3 hours. Let all smoked salmon sit overnight to finish curing for best eating results.

GRILLED HALIBUT STEAKS
WITH TWO SAUCE CHOICES AND TWO FLAVORED BUTTER CHOICES

INGREDIENTS:

- 4 lbs. 1-inch halibut steaks
- ¼ c. olive oil
- the Galley Wench's Smoked Salt or kosher salt to taste
- fresh ground pepper to taste

DIRECTIONS:

TO MAKE THE FISH: Pat the fish dry with paper towels. Rub the fish with the oil. Sprinkle with the salt & pepper. Grill on high 2 or 3 minutes per side for a 1-inch steak.

Sauce #1 - Mediterranean style

INGREDIENTS:

- 1 stick melted butter
- 6 cloves garlic, minced
- zest of one lemon
- 1 c. sliced scallions
- ½ c. pitted kalamata olives, sliced
- 1 c. medium diced tomatoes
- 1 c. chopped marinated artichoke hearts (packed in olive oil are better)
- juice of one lemon
- ¼ c. white wine

DIRECTIONS:

Melt the butter in a skillet. Sauté the garlic until soft. Add the remaining ingredients except for the scallions and the tomatoes. Simmer sauce about 10 minutes. Pour over halibut steaks, garnish with diced tomatoes and sliced scallions, and serve.

Sauce #2 - Lemon pepper style, the Wench way

INGREDIENTS:

- zest of 6 lemons
- 1 cube of butter
- 1 bulb of garlic (not a clove), coarsely chopped
- Galley Wench's Smoked Salt or kosher salt
- 1 c. finely chopped parsley
- ½ tsp. cayenne pepper (optional but yummy)
- wedges of fresh lemon
- ¼ c. fresh lemon juice
- ¼ c. sherry

DIRECTIONS:

Melt the butter in a skillet, add the garlic, and cook on a medium-low heat until caramelized. Add lemon zest, black pepper, and cayenne to the garlic & butter. Add the lemon juice, and cook simmering 10 to 15 minutes until it is good and hot. Pour sauce over fish, and garnish with a sprinkle of the parsley and lemon wedges. (Chopped capers would be a nice option also if you are fond of them.)

Italian Flavors Seasoned Butter

INGREDIENTS:

- 1 lb. butter, room temperature (soft)
- 1 fire-roasted and peeled red pepper, diced and chilled
- 1 c. diced sun-dried tomatoes (the kind in olive oil)
- 1 bulb roasted garlic, peeled, diced, and chilled
- zest of 1 lemon
- ¼ c. chopped fresh basil
- 2 tbsp. chopped fresh oregano
- 2 tbsp. chopped Italian parsley
- Galley Wench's Smoked Salt or kosher salt
- fresh ground pepper

DIRECTIONS:

In a large bowl, whip all the ingredients into the butter. Spoon butter mixture onto plastic wrap, roll into a log or place it into a zipper baggie, and press it flat after it is sealed. Chill butter until firm and cut into pieces. Before using the butter, remove from refrigerator, and let warm at room temperature to soften.

Pistachio Butter

INGREDIENTS:

- 1 c. firmly packed light brown sugar
- 1 lb. butter room temperature (soft)
- ¼ c. pistachio nut oil
- 1 c. shelled chopped pistachios

DIRECTIONS:

Whip the brown sugar and butter until fluffy. Slowly add the pistachio nut oil to the butter, and continue to whip until completely incorporated. Fold in toasted pistachios. Spoon butter mixture onto plastic wrap, roll into a log or place it into a zipper baggie, and press it flat and about 2 inches thick after it is sealed. Chill butter until firm, and cut into pieces. Before using the butter, remove from refrigerator, and let warm at room temperature to soften.

Pink Peppercorn & Orange-Crusted Salmon Medallions with Miso Caesar

INGREDIENTS:

- 2 fillets salmon, skinned and boned
- zest of one orange
- ½ c. coarsely ground pink peppercorns
- kosher salt
- 2 tbsp. peanut oil
- ½ c. mayo
- 1 tbsp. yellow miso
- 2½ tsp. fish sauce
- 1 tbsp. lemon juice
- 2 heads romaine, torn in bite-size pieces
- 1½ c. croutons
- ½ c. shredded Romano cheese
- 6 lemon & 6 orange wedges

DIRECTIONS:

Using a round cutter (cookie cutter, biscuit cutter), cut out 18 medallions from the salmon fillets. Sprinkle the salmon lightly with the salt. In a small bowl combine the orange zest and the peppercorns. Press one side of the salmon medallion into the pepper/zest mixture. Heat a skillet and the peanut oil to medium hot. Sear first the side of the salmon that does not have the peppercorns on it about 2 to 3 minutes. Reduce heat to low, turn over the salmon medallions, cook another 2 to 3 minutes, and remove from heat and set aside. In a small bowl combine the mayo, miso, fish sauce, and lemon juice. In a large bowl add the romaine, and toss with the dressing. Add the croutons and Romano cheese. Place salad in the center of serving dish, place 3 salmon medallions on the top of each salad, and serve garnished with a lemon and an orange wedge.

You can make your own croutons very easily by melting a little butter with a clove of garlic and tossing it in some stale bread cut into cubes and toasting it lightly in a 350-degree oven.

Rabbit Fricassee

INGREDIENTS:

- 2 rabbits, both cut into 5 pieces
- 4 slices thick fatty bacon
- ½ can all natural apple juice concentrate
- 2 c. water
- 1 c. cream
- ¼ c. fresh tarragon finely chopped
- 2 tbsp. raw sugar
- salt & freshly ground pepper

DIRECTIONS:

In a large Dutch oven, cook the bacon until all fat has rendered and the bacon is crispy. Set aside bacon for another preparation. Generously salt and pepper the rabbit meat. Heat the bacon drippings until smoking hot.

Sear the rabbit on both sides. Once the rabbit has nicely browned, add the apple juice concentrate and water. Cover and bake in a 320-degree oven for 1½ hours or until the rabbit is fork-tender.

Remove the rabbit meat carefully to a plate and tent with foil to keep meat warm and moist. Heat pan juices in Dutch oven over high heat, whisking occasionally until they reduce and start to thicken. Add heavy cream and continue to cook until the mixture becomes a beautiful and thick golden sauce. Remove from heat. Season with sugar, and add salt and pepper to taste. Stir the tarragon into the sauce just before serving. Before serving, ladle sauce over rabbit.

Ultimate Crab Royal

INGREDIENTS:

- 3 lbs. king crab legs, split
- ½ c. butter
- 2 tbsp. fish sauce or to taste
- 1 tbsp. garlic chili paste or to taste (spicy)
- ½ c. fresh chopped scallions
- ½ c. dry vermouth
- 1 c. melted butter
- 1 tbsp. fish sauce
- 2 tsp. garlic chili sauce

DIRECTIONS:

In a very large pot that has a tight-fitting lid, melt the butter. As soon as the butter begins to foam, add the crab and toss in the butter. As the crab begins to sizzle well, add to the pot the fish sauce, garlic chili paste, scallions, and vermouth. Cover with lid, and let steam about 5 minutes just to heat crab through and cook off the alcohol in the vermouth. Remove from heat, and transfer to a large serving dish, broth and all.

If you need additional butter for dipping the crab in, melt butter, and add a bit of fish sauce and garlic chili paste to it. But the broth will be to die for.

My favorite way to serve it is with one of those good crusty artisan breads. I would like sourdough best, but it would have to be really crusty, even a little stale so it will hold up when you are dunking it in the broth.

My favorite drink with such a dish is a good crispy cold ale to fill my tankard with. Make sure your ale is one that is not too bitter, or you will not taste the crab.

Moose Scallopini

INGREDIENTS:

- 2 lbs. moose backstrap or tenderloin, sliced ¼-inch thickness and flattened
- olive oil and 2 tbsp. butter for frying
- ½ c. flour
- ¼ c. finely diced shallots
- 1½ tbsp. finely diced garlic
- 1½ c. sliced cremini mushrooms
- ¼ c. lemon juice
- ¼ c. Chianti (dry red table wine)
- kosher salt & freshly ground pepper
- 1 c. seeded and diced fresh Roma tomato
- ¼ c. finely chopped fresh Italian parsley
- salt & pepper

DIRECTIONS:

Heat oil and butter on medium high heat in a nice big skillet. Season the moose with salt & pepper, and lightly dredge in the flour. Sauté moose in the butter/oil until light golden in color, taking care not to cook it too hot so as not to scorch the flour and turn it bitter. After browning, reserve meat to a warm plate. When all your moose is brown and on the plate, add a bit more butter and oil to your pan, heat just until the butter is melted and starts to bubble, then add the shallots and garlic, giving it a quick stir. Then add to that the mushrooms, and sauté them until they are starting to brown. Return moose meat to the pan, and pour over the wine and lemon juice. Cook about 15 minutes or until the alcohol has dissipated. Remove meat to a warm serving dish, and turn up the heat on the skillet. Reduce liquid remaining in the pan by half, and remove from heat. For added richness and flavor at this point, you can add another tablespoon of butter to the sauce, stirring until melted into the sauce. Taste and see if it needs salt or pepper. Pour over the moose meat. Sprinkle the diced tomato and parsley over the top, and garnish with wedges of lemon and serve.

Coconut Halibut

INGREDIENTS:

- 3 lbs. halibut, cut into thick strips 3 inches thick and about 4 inches long
- Fat for frying, duck fat, peanut oil, or lard
- 3 c. panko breading
- 2 c. shredded coconut
- 1 c. buttermilk
- 3 egg whites
- 1 c. flour or more for first coating of the fish

DIRECTIONS:

Mix panko and coconut together, beat together buttermilk and egg whites, coat halibut chunks with flour, dredge them in the buttermilk mixture, roll them in the panko/coconut, and place on a baking sheet in a single layer. Place the fish in the freezer for an hour to help it dry out a bit. This trick helps to keep the coating intact also, and it seems to get a little less greasy to me. Fry a few chunks at a time, being careful not to do too many at once, or it reduces the heat of your oil and slows the cooking, which causes your fish to get greasy. The fish will be cooked just as soon as it turns a nice golden brown. I like to drain excess oil off the fish by placing it on a rack with a paper towel under it. This keeps your coating from getting soggy as fast. It is always best to keep your coating extra crispy. Serve while nice and hot.

Root Beer-Glazed Plank Roasted Salmon

INGREDIENTS:

- Ingredients:
- 3 lbs. salmon fillet
- ¼ c. freshly toasted ground black pepper
- salt
- cottonwood, birch, or cedar planks
- 2 Henry Weinhard's root beers or other high-quality natural ingredients root beers that you love. (Since it will be reduced into a sauce, it's very important that it's good quality and natural ingredients. Artificial ingredients make for a terrible sauce when they get concentrated by reducing.)

DIRECTIONS:

In a saucepan pour in both root beers. Cook at a medium-low heat at a light simmer until reduced and thick like a syrup. Keep an eye on it so it doesn't bubble over or cook too slowly, or you will be at it for a long time.

Preheat oven and plank to 375 degrees. Season the salmon on both sides with the salt & toasted pepper. Place salmon fillet in center of plank. Place plank on a baking sheet, and bake for 15 minutes.

Brush with glaze. Bake an additional 5 minutes, just long enough to cook the glaze into the fish. Serves 4–6.

Turkey à la King

INGREDIENTS:

- 2 c. leftover turkey or brown fresh raw turkey breast or thigh meat, medium diced
- ½ medium-sized red onion, sliced thin
- ½ red sweet bell pepper, sliced thin
- ½ green bell pepper, sliced thin
- 3 tbsp. butter
- kosher salt & white pepper
- béchamel sauce:
- ¼ c. unsalted butter
- ¼ c. all-purpose unbleached flour
- 2½ c. scalded cream or half & half
- 1 small onion studded with 2 cloves
- salt & nutmeg to taste

DIRECTIONS:

Melt butter with the oil on medium heat. Season the turkey with the salt & white pepper. Sauté the turkey until heated and starting to turn a lightly golden brown. This will not take very long, and care needs to be taken so as not to cook it too much if it's leftovers and precooked, because it can dry out. If using raw, cook it through. Remove turkey to a warm plate. In the same pan, while it is still hot, add the peppers and onions. Cook until wilted but not caramelized. Add turkey back to skillet, and pour over béchamel sauce. Taste for seasoning. Simmer on medium-low heat until bubbly for 5 minutes and serve.

TO MAKE SAUCE: Add cream to a saucepan, bring just under a boil on medium heat while stirring, and set aside. Melt butter until it just starts to foam, and add the flour, stirring until it is combined with the melted butter. Cook over medium-low heat for 2 minutes, making a light roux. Stir scalded cream slowly into the roux, and simmer until it starts to thicken. Add studded onion, and simmer about 20 minutes, keeping it stirred. Strain and reserve.

The Galley Wench's Basic Stuffing Recipe

INGREDIENTS:

- 8 c. bread, cubed, dried, and toasted
- 1 large onion, medium diced
- 1 c. celery, medium diced
- 2 c. sliced mushrooms
- 1 bulb garlic, peeled and diced
- 2 eggs
- ½ c. butter
- 2 tbsp. fresh chopped sage
- 1½ to 2 c. broth

DIRECTIONS:

Melt butter in a large sauté pan, add vegetables, and cook on medium-low heat until caramelized. Toss caramelized vegetable and butter mixture with the dried toasted bread cubes, sage, and eggs. Gradually add broth, tossing to coat the bread evenly, using less broth if you plan to put it in a bird and more broth if you plan to bake it separately. If baked separately, do so in a 350-degree oven for 25 to 30 minutes if in a bird, then bake until stuffing reaches 160 degrees.

Wench's Famous Salmon Patties

INGREDIENTS:

- 1 lb. fresh salmon, small diced, or 1-pt. jar of canned salmon, drained
- 2 slices white bread
- Alaskan Amber Beer
- 1 medium onion, small diced
- 1 large egg
- 3 cloves garlic, minced
- 2 tbsp. Italian parsley, finely chopped
- salt & pepper to taste
- duck fat or grapeseed oil for frying

DIRECTIONS:

In a medium bowl soak the bread with enough Alaskan Amber to make it wet but not sopping. Into the bowl add the fish, onion, garlic, parsley, and salt & pepper to taste. Mix thoroughly so everything is evenly distributed. Using ⅓ cup dried measuring cup, scoop out fish mixture. Form a ball, then flatten into patties. Continue with the rest of the fish mixture. Heat oil in a skillet on medium heat. Fry the patties until golden on each side (about 5 minutes). Be careful not to crowd the pan. Drain on paper towels and serve.

Alaskan Spruce Tip Shrimp

INGREDIENTS:

- 3 lbs. peeled large Alaska shrimp
- ¼ c. yellow mustard
- 2 tbsp. mayonnaise
- 2 cloves grated garlic
- ½ tsp. fresh lime zest
- 1 tsp. fresh dill, finely chopped
- 1 tbsp. spruce tips, finely chopped
- 1 tbsp. fresh lime juice
- 1 tbsp. fish sauce
- salt & pepper to taste
- skewers

DIRECTIONS:

In a small bowl combine the mustard, mayo, garlic, lime zest, dill, spruce tips, lime juice, and fish sauce. Mix well until evenly combined, and salt & pepper to taste if needed. Pour marinade over shrimp, and stir them until well coated. Let soak 30 minutes to 1 hour in the refrigerator. Skewer shrimp 6 to a stick. Reserve the remaining marinade for basting. Grill or broil the fish over medium-high heat, turning often and basting after each turn. Just as the shrimp begin to curl, remove from heat and serve.

Bacon-Wrapped Basil Halibut

INGREDIENTS:

- 2 lbs. halibut cut in 2-inch x 4-inch chunks, enough to make 8 pieces
- 8 slices of fatty bacon
- 8 large basil leaves
- 2 tsp. lemon zest
- 2½ tbsp. celery salt
- 2 tsp. MSG
- 1 tsp. fresh ground green peppercorns

DIRECTIONS:

In a large skillet on low heat, render much of the fat from the bacon. Cook the bacon until done and tender but not brown. Set aside the bacon to cool, and reserve the pan with the bacon fat to cook the fish in. In a small bowl mix together the celery salt, MSG, green pepper, and lemon zest. Liberally season all the sides of the halibut with the seasoning mix, and pat it into the fish well. Lay two basil leaves on the flattest side of the halibut. Wind a slice of bacon around the fish with the basil on it. Secure both ends of the bacon with toothpicks. Repeat with the rest of the fish. Get the pan with the bacon fat in it very hot. Carefully place each halibut piece basil side down in the skillet. Sear for 2 minutes on one side or until the bacon becomes golden. Turn over and do the same on the other side. Turn off the heat and remove it from the heat. Place the butter in the pan and, as it melts, baste the fish with the butter. Once the fish is nicely basted, remove it from the heat to a plate, and allow it to rest 5 minutes before serving.

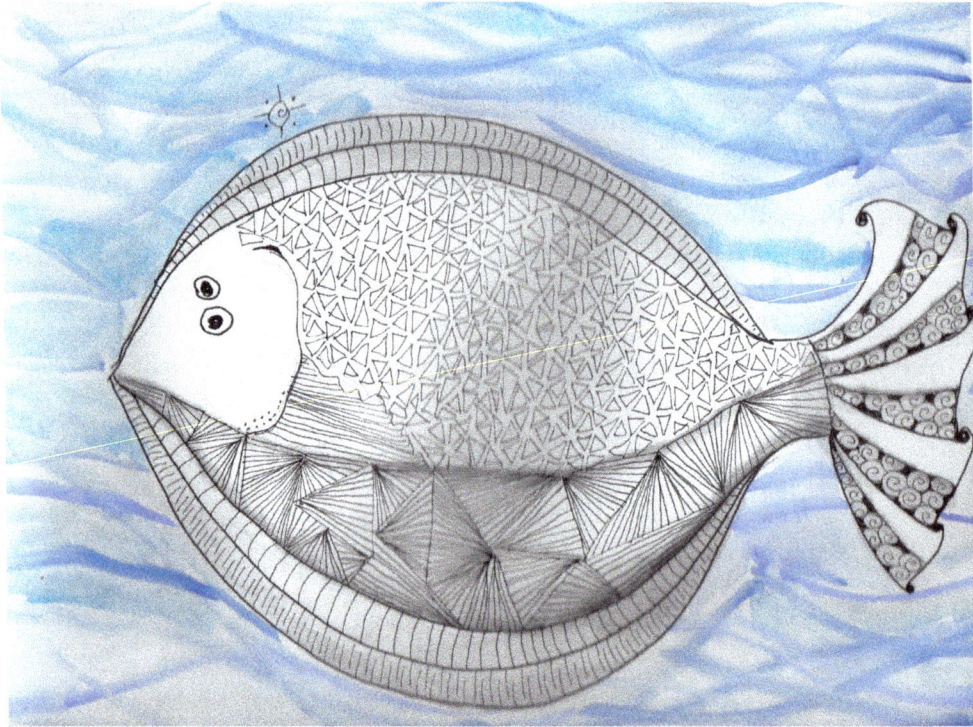

Galley Wench's Own Fry Bread

INGREDIENTS:

- 1 duck egg
- 1 c. whole milk, warmed up
- ⅓ c. melted duck fat
- 1 tsp. popcorn salt
- 2 tbsp. raw sugar
- 3 tbsp. baking powder
- 2 c. high-gluten bread flour
- 2 c. all-purpose unbleached flour
- enough oil in a cast-iron skillet for the bread to float

DIRECTIONS:

Before you start, take a deep breath. Slowly let the breath out, and let go of any negative thoughts. Slowly take in another deep breath, bring in loving and happy thoughts with it. Now you're ready to begin.

In a large bowl sift or whisk together the dry ingredients, making a well in the center for the wet ingredients. Vigorously whisk the wet ingredients until very foamy. Pour the wet ingredients into the well made in the dry ingredients. Mix thoroughly by hand until it comes together as a dough. Continue to knead the dough until even though it is sticky, it no longer sticks to your hands (roughly 10 minutes or 4 good songs). Pull off handfuls of dough, and roll it into balls. Cover lightly and allow to rest 20 minutes. Heat oil for frying to 350 degrees. Flatten dough balls to about ¼ inch thick either with your hands or with a rolling pin. Gently lay flattened dough in the hot oil in the direction away from you. Fry both sides until perfectly golden brown. Drain finished fry bread on paper towels. Serve immediately while it's still nice and warm.

Red Salmon Mac & Cheese

INGREDIENTS:

- 1 lb. gently poached red salmon broken up into large flakes
- ⅓ c. fresh peas
- ¼ c. finely sliced green onion
- ¼ c. unbleached all-purpose flour
- ¼ c. butter
- ½ c. whole milk
- ½ c. half & half
- ½ c. heavy cream
- ⅓ c. grated Pecorino Romano
- ⅓ c. Havarti, small dice
- ⅓ c. whole milk mozzarella, small dice
- 2 boxes Kraft Macaroni and Cheese

DIRECTIONS:

Cook pasta in salted water 5 minutes, add the green peas, cook for 2 minutes, and then drain. In the pot you cooked the pasta in, melt the butter, and combine it with the flour. Cook the butter and flour on medium-low heat for 2 minutes while stirring constantly. Do not allow it to brown. Add the powder from the mac & cheese, and whisk it together with the butter flour mixture. Add the milk, half & half, heavy cream, cheese, and pasta all at once back into the pot. Stir gently so the bottom does not scorch until it is hot and the cheese is melted. Gently fold in the flaked salmon. Garnish the top with the green onion, and serve right away while the sauce is creamy and smooth.

Honey Mustard Pork Chops

INGREDIENTS:

- 4 1½-inch bone-in pork chops, well marbled
- chef salt (equal parts salt, sugar, and MSG, lightly flecked with toasted freshly ground pepper)
- 1 c. unbleached all-purpose flour
- 4 cloves garlic, grated
- 3 c. strong mustard
- ¼ c. honey
- 2 tbsp. fresh tarragon, chopped
- 1 tsp. fresh thyme leaves
- 1 tsp. salt, 1¼ tsp. toasted fresh ground peppercorns
- 4 c. coarse breadcrumbs
- 1 stick of butter
- ½ c. mustard oil

DIRECTIONS:

Season the pork chops, including the bone, generously with the chef salt mixture. Allow the pork chops to sit seasoned while you prepare the rest of the ingredients. In 3 dishes big enough to fit a pork chop in, prepare a coating station. In the first dish add flour. In the second dish combine the mustard, garlic, honey, tarragon and thyme leaves, salt & pepper, whisk together to combine evenly. In the third dish add the breadcrumbs. To bread the pork chops, first press flour into the pork chop firmly until well coated, shake off excess. Then dredge in the honey mustard mixture until evenly coated, then into the breadcrumbs, pressing firmly into the pork chop. Repeat with the other pork chops, and lay each one on a baking sheet. Place the pork chops on the baking sheet into a freezer for 10 to 15 minutes to help coating adhere to the pork chops. While the pork chops chill, warm the butter and mustard oil slowly until butter is finished foaming, but don't allow it to brown too much. Brown the pork chops uniformly on both sides until crispy and cooked through on medium heat 15 to 20 minutes.

MOOSE SPAGHETTI

INGREDIENTS:

- 3 lbs. ground moose meat (can use buffalo instead)
- 2 tsp. baking soda dissolved in ¼ c. of cold water
- 1 c. salt pork
- 3 sticks celery, large dice
- 1 whole carrot, large dice
- 1 large onion, large dice
- 1 red bell pepper
- 1 bulb of garlic, peeled
- ½ lb. cremini or portobello mushroom, large dice
- 2 1-lb. cans of Italian San Marzano tomatoes, crushed by hand
- ¼ c. Italian tomato paste
- 1 c. red wine
- 1 tbsp. crushed dried oregano
- 2 tbsp. sugar
- pinch of crushed red pepper
- 1 small bunch of fresh thyme
- salt & pepper to taste

DIRECTIONS:

Mix the water and baking soda mixture into the moose meat, and let it set as you prepare the rest of the ingredients. In a food processor, pulse the salt pork until coarsely chopped. Add the garlic and vegetables, and pulse until the mixture becomes a paste. Cook the paste with the oregano and red pepper flakes in a large heave pot until cooked through and starting to brown. Add the tomato paste, and continue cooking until it starts to brown again but not too dark. Add the moose meat, and cook just until it's no longer red. Add the tomatoes into the pot, rinse out the tomato container with the wine, and pour it into the pot. Season with the sugar, salt & pepper, and the bunch of fresh thyme. Simmer gently 30 to 45 minutes, stirring frequently. Serve with your favorite hearty pasta.

Wine-Baked Silver Salmon

INGREDIENTS:

- 4 8-oz. sections of silver salmon fillet
- salt & fresh ground pepper
- 2 tbsp. clarified butter
- 1 c. dry vermouth or very dry white wine
- 1 tbsp. fish sauce
- 4 tbsp. butter
- ¼ c. parsley, finely chopped
- ¼ c. green onion, finely sliced
- 4 cloves fresh garlic, minced
- 1 tsp. minced capers
- 8 lemon wedges, seeded
- additional salt & pepper to taste

DIRECTIONS:

Salt and pepper the salmon fillet sections generously. Heat clarified butter in a cast-iron skillet or other heavy pan. As soon as the butter is hot, place salmon skin side down, and cook until the skin is brown and crispy, but the fish is not cooked much. Remove the salmon to a plate with the skin side up. In the pan you browned the salmon in, add the garlic and capers, and cook briefly until fragrant. Add the wine and the fish sauce, and heat just until it starts to simmer. Carefully place the fish back in the pan skin side up. Place a tbsp. of butter on top of each fillet. Transfer the pan with the fish in the wine into a 420-degree oven. Cook for 10 minutes. Remove from the oven. Transfer the fish to a plate to rest 5 to 10 minutes. Return the pan to the heat, and keep it warm. Just before serving, stir the parsley and green onion into the pan sauce. Spoon pan sauce onto plate or bowl, then place the salmon on top so the skin stays crispy. Serve.

Moose Burgers

INGREDIENTS:

- 2 lbs. ground moose meat (80 to 85% lean with 15 to 20% fat ratio)
- 2 tbsp. shallot, finely chopped
- ½ c. cremini mushrooms, finely chopped
- 2 tbsp. butter
- 1 tsp. baking soda dissolved in 3 tbsp. mushroom soy sauce
- ¼ tsp. red pepper flake
- salt & fresh ground pepper

DIRECTIONS:

In a heavy skillet melt the butter. Sweat the mushrooms and the shallots in the butter until they just start to brown. Set aside to cool to room temperature. In a bowl add the moose burger. Sprinkle over the meat the baking soda, mushroom soy sauce mix. Add the mushroom shallot mixture, red pepper flakes. Mix the meat mixture to combine all the ingredients evenly. Add salt & pepper to your taste. Do the mixing gently, and don't overwork the mixture, or it will become tough. Divide the meat into four equal ½ lbs. Form into balls, then flatten to shape into patties. Cook on a fire, grill, or butter a cast-iron pan or griddle. Cook 5 minutes on each side since they will be nice big patties for nice medium rare. Cook longer if you want less pink in the middle, cook less if you like more rare. You can add cheese or any of your favorite toppings. Tastes perfect on its own with only a bun, on a bun with the works, or even without a bun with a salad.

Galley Wench Style Menudo

INGREDIENTS:

- 4 pig feet
- 4 pig tails
- 3 lbs. honeycomb tripe, large dice
- 4 large onions
- 1 gallon light stock (pork, chicken, veal)
- 3 2-lb. cans of hominy, drained (white or yellow)
- 4 large bay leaves
- 6 dried ancho peppers
- 1 bulb of garlic, left whole
- 4 large ripe tomatoes, large dice
- 4 large poblano peppers, large dice
- 1 tbsp. MSG
- salt & fresh ground pepper to taste
- fresh cilantro, lime wedges, sliced serrano peppers (optional for garnish)

DIRECTIONS:

In a very large soup pot sweat onions just until they start to change color. Add pigs' feet, tails, tripe, hominy, bay leaves, dried ancho, whole bulb of garlic (unpeeled), stock, MSG, and salt & pepper. Bring to a rolling boil for 10 minutes. Reduce heat to a very slow simmer. Put on a lid and cook very low and slow for 4 hours until the tails, feet, and tripe are tender. Add more stock or water if it is reducing too much. After cooked well, remove the bulb of garlic to cool. Add the tomatoes and fresh poblano peppers the last 30 minutes of cooking. Taste for seasoning and adjust with salt & pepper if needed. Squeeze the garlic out of the paper and stir it back into the soup. Serve hot with garnishes on the side (optional).

WHOLE ROASTED PIG HEAD

INGREDIENTS:

- 1 whole pig head (brains removed)
- 1 750 ml. bottle white wine
- water to cover
- 1 c. sugar
- 1 c. honey
- ¼ c. salt
- 2 carrots, 2 celery stumps, 2 bunches parsley stems, peels from 4 large onions
- 1 whole bulb of fresh garlic, unpeeled
- ¼ c. fresh ginger, large dice
- 1 tsp. whole cloves
- 1 tbsp. whole peppercorns
- 4 star anise
- 4 large bay leaves
- butter
- small apple

DIRECTIONS:

In a large pot with a lid and plenty of room for the pig's head, place the pig's head in the bottom. Add everything to the pot except the butter. Bring to a full boil for 10 minutes. Skim the foam that comes to the top and discard. Reduce heat to low simmer. Cook 6 to 8 hours until the ears and snout are tender. Allow to cool totally in the broth. Remove the head from the broth (strain the broth and freeze for soup or bean making). Dry the head thoroughly. Place pig's head in a large roasting pan with apple in its mouth. Brush all over with melted butter and roast in a 350-degree oven 30 to 45 minutes, basting with butter halfway through. Soon as the pig head has browned and gotten crispy, remove from oven and onto waiting platter. Serve hot.

Honey-Glazed Smoked Duck

INGREDIENTS:

- 1 duck
- 2 gal. cold water
- 4 c. honey
- 1 c. raw sugar
- 1 c. salt
- ¼ c. baking soda
- ½ c. honey
- 1 stick of butter, melted
- 1 tsp. freshly ground black pepper

DIRECTIONS:

Remove giblets and/or sauce packet from the duck if it has it. Poke the duck all over with the tip of a sharp knife (specially on the breast). Combine the cold water, honey, sugar, salt, and baking soda in a large container that will fit in the fridge. Stir together until everything is dissolved completely, making sure nothing is left settled on the bottom. Submerge the duck in the brine using something with some weight to keep it covered completely by the brine. Let sit 24 to 48 hours in the brine. Remove from brine and drain completely, patting dry with paper towels, and allow to sit in the fridge uncovered until the skin becomes completely dry. Get smoker going and place duck in. Smoke 1 hour for hot smoker, 3 hours for cold smoker. Dissolve the honey in the melted butter and black pepper and keep it whisked and emulsified. Remove duck from smoker to a roasting pan. Brush all over generously with the honey butter. Roast in a 325-degree oven slowly for 45 minutes, basting occasionally with the honey butter. Remove from oven and rest on serving platter 20 minutes before cutting into it. Slice and serve.

Moose Meatloaf

INGREDIENTS:

- 3 lbs. ground moose meat (85% lean, 15% fat)
- 3 slices white bread soaked with heavy cream
- 1 medium onion, very finely chopped
- 1 carrot, finely chopped
- 2 stalks celery, finely chopped
- 2 duck eggs
- 6 cloves fresh garlic, finely minced
- ¼ c. soy sauce with 2 tsp. baking soda dissolved in it
- 2 tsp. Worcestershire sauce
- ¼ c. cornstarch
- ¼ c. fresh parsley, freshly chopped
- salt & freshly cracked pepper to taste
- 3 tbsp. butter
- ¾ c. ketchup, 1 tsp. dry mustard mixed with 1 tbsp. brown sugar, mixed thoroughly until sugar is dissolved

DIRECTIONS:

In a big enough skillet place butter and chopped vegetables. Cook until soft and starting to caramelize. Set aside to cool to room temperature. In a large bowl add the moose meat. Mix in the soy sauce/baking soda mixture, sautéed cooled vegetables, eggs, bread, garlic, Worcestershire sauce, cornstarch, and parsley. Mix very well so all the ingredients are evenly distributed. Salt & pepper to desired taste and mix well again. Be careful not to overwork the meat mixture, so be gentle or it will get tough. Bake at 350 degrees for 1 hour. Remove from heat and spread the ketchup mixture over the top. Put back in the oven for another 20 minutes until the sauce is cooked onto the meat and thickens slightly. Remove from the oven and allow to cool for 30 minutes, or it will fall apart when you try to slice it. Drain well, slice, and serve.

The Best Chicken Feet Snack Ever

INGREDIENTS:

- 4 lbs. prepared chicken feet (nails and outer skin removed)
- water to cover
- 1 c. raw sugar
- 1 c. soy sauce
- 2 tbsp. salt, 1 tsp. baking soda
- 1 c. plum sauce
- 2 tbsp. fish sauce
- 1 tsp. MSG
- juice of ½ lime
- 2 tsp. sambal chili sauce, 1 tsp. Thai hot pepper flakes
- ¼ c. raw or brown sugar

DIRECTIONS:

In a big pot add chicken feet and cover with water. To the pot add the raw sugar, soy sauce, salt, and baking soda. Bring to a rolling boil and skim off and discard any foam that rises to the top. Put a lid on and reduce heat to a slow simmer. Cook 45 minutes to 1 hour or until the chicken feet are very tender. Cool them in the broth until they can be handled. Drain the chicken feet and allow them to dry (save the cooking liquid to use as chicken broth). In a bowl, mix together the plum sauce, fish sauce, MSG, lime juice, chili sauce, pepper flakes, and brown sugar until dissolved. Toss the chicken feet in half of the sauce. Spread out on a baking sheet and roast until the chicken feet brown nicely. Remove from the oven and carefully toss while hot in the rest of the sauce. Serve with plenty of napkins.

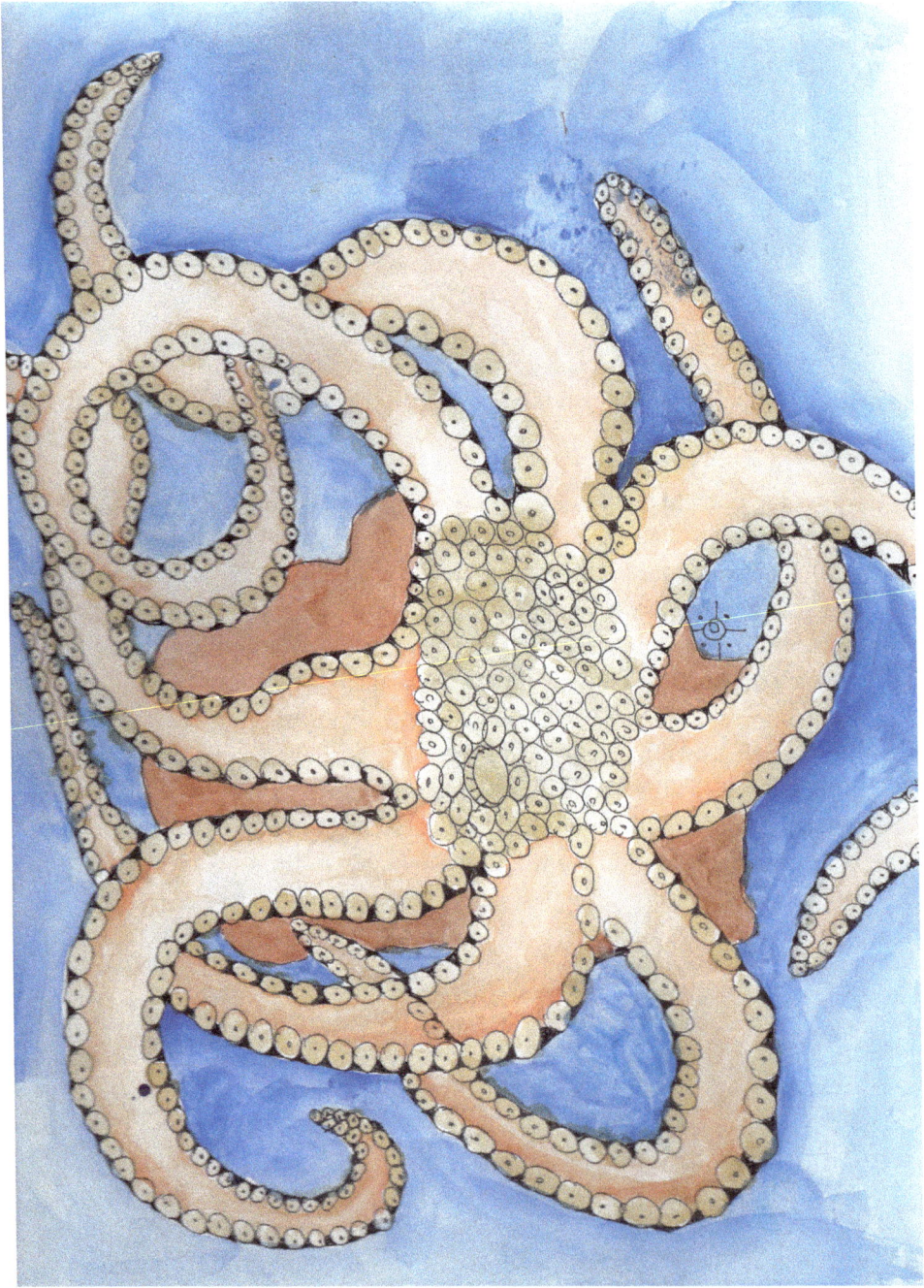

Pasta Salad with Alaska Spot Shrimp

INGREDIENTS:

- 1 box good quality fusilli pasta (cooked according to package directions, drained and rinsed with cold water until chilled)
- 2 lbs. large Alaska spot shrimp (poached for 3 minutes in a court bouillon, drained, chilled in cold water, peeled and deveined)
- 1½ c. pickled dill green beans, large dice (pickled okra or asparagus can substitute)
- 1 c. black olives, cut in half crossways
- 1½ c. cherry tomatoes, halved
- 1½ c. fresh shelled peas (thawed frozen can substitute)
- 1 c. fresh cauliflower, cut into small sections
- 1 c. chopped marinated artichoke hearts
- ½ c. fresh parsley, finely chopped
- ½ c. green onion, finely chopped
- 2 tbsp. capers, finely chopped
- juice & zest of 2 lemons
- ½ c. good olive oil
- 1 tsp. seedy brown mustard
- 1 clove grated garlic
- 1 tsp. fish sauce
- salt & fresh ground pepper to taste

DIRECTIONS:

In a large bowl, combine all ingredients thoroughly so evenly combined. Chill for 1 hour; can be made the night before. Serve.

PURPLE POTATO SALAD

INGREDIENTS:

- 6 purple baking potatoes, baked 45 minutes, chilled, medium dice (red potatoes or Yukon gold can be substituted)
- 6 boiled duck eggs (peeled, large dice)
- 1 large onion, sliced thickly into rings, blanched, medium dice
- 1 tbsp. capers, chopped
- ¼ c. fresh parsley, finely chopped
- ¼ c. fresh dill, finely chopped
- 1 tsp. fresh thyme leaves
- 1 c. green olives with pimentos, sliced
- 1 c. mayo
- 1 c. crème fraiche
- 1 tbsp. fish sauce
- 1 tbsp. horseradish sauce
- juice and zest of 1 lemon
- 2 tsp. celery salt
- 1 tsp. dry mustard
- salt & pepper to taste

DIRECTIONS:

In a large bowl, layer potatoes, eggs, onion, capers, herbs, and olives. Season with the celery salt and salt & pepper to taste by tossing lightly. In a separate bowl, make the dressing by combining the mayo, crème fraiche, fish sauce, horseradish, lemon juice and zest, and dry mustard. Mix thoroughly. Pour dressing over potato mixture and toss lightly. Taste again for seasoning. Allow to rest in the refrigerator at least 1 hour. Can be made the day before. Serve.

Egg Salad

INGREDIENTS:

- 8 duck eggs (boiled, chilled, peeled), large dice
- ¼ c. fresh chives, finely chopped
- ¼ c. peppadew peppers, finely chopped
- 1 tsp. truffle oil
- ¼ c. mayo
- 2 tbsp. crème fraiche
- salt & freshly ground pepper to taste

DIRECTIONS:

In a medium bowl, layer the eggs, chives, and peppadew peppers. In another bowl, make the dressing, whisk together the truffle oil, mayo, and crème fraiche. Pour the dressing over the egg mixture. Toss lightly until evenly combined. Adjust seasoning to taste with salt & pepper. Serve.

DEVILED EGGS

INGREDIENTS:

- 1 dozen duck eggs (boiled and peeled), halved, yolks separated into a bowl
- 1 tbsp. truffle oil
- ¼ c. mayo
- 1 tsp. truffle salt
- 12 slices bread-and-butter pickles, finely diced
- pastry bag with large star tip

DIRECTIONS:

On a platter big enough, place egg whites in neat rows. In the bowl of egg yolks add the truffle oil and mayo. With a hand mixer, beat mixture until light and fluffy with no lumps. Fill the pastry bag with the egg yolk mixture. Fill each egg white with enough yolk to fill the hole generously. Sprinkle a light dusting of truffle salt over each egg. Spoon a little diced bread-and-butter pickle on the top of each egg to garnish. Serve right away or make ahead of time, up to the day before. If made ahead of time, cover and refrigerate; bring out 30 minutes ahead of time to take the chill off before serving.

Moose Heart Tacos

INGREDIENTS:

- 1 to 2 lbs. moose heart, sinew and gristle removed, sliced ½-inch slices (beef heart can substitute)
- 1 shot tequila
- ¼ c. olive oil
- zest of 1 lime
- 4 cloves of garlic, minced fine
- salt & freshly ground pepper to taste
- 2 c. fresh arugula
- 2 large ripe tomatoes
- 2 thick slices sweet onion
- 2 tomatillos, halved
- 3 cloves garlic, unpeeled
- ¼ c. ancho peppers in adobo
- ½ c. fresh cilantro, chopped
- juice of 1 lime
- corn tortillas, lightly toasted

DIRECTIONS:

Mix well in a bowl the tequila, olive oil, lime zest, minced garlic, and salt & pepper. Toss the heart meat thoroughly to evenly coat. Chill for 1 hour or overnight. Make the sauce by browning the tomato, onion, unpeeled garlic, and tomatillos in a hot cast-iron pan. In a blender, combine browned veggies with the ancho peppers in adobo, cilantro, and lime juice. Blend until a smooth sauce, taste for seasoning, and add salt & pepper if needed (sauce can be made the night before and stored in the refrigerator). Sear the heart meat quickly, 2 to 3 minutes on each side. On a hot tortilla layer arugula and heart, top with sauce, and serve.

Pork Belly

INGREDIENTS:

- 3 lbs. pork belly, cut into 3-inch x 3-inch-thick slices
- large pot with steamer racks
- 4 c. water
- 1 c. soy sauce
- 1 tsp. clove
- 1 tbsp. black peppercorns
- 4 star anise
- 1 tbsp. maple extract
- ½ c. maple syrup
- ¼ c. raw sugar
- 2 tbsp. soy sauce
- 1 tsp. fresh grated ginger
- 1 tsp. fresh grated garlic
- ½ tsp. MSG
- salt & freshly ground pepper to taste

DIRECTIONS:

In a jar with a tight-fitting lid, combine the maple syrup, raw sugar, 2 tbsp. soy sauce, ginger, garlic, and MSG. Make sure the lid is on tight and shake until sugar is completely dissolved. Set aside so the flavors can combine while you prepare the pork belly.

In a large pot, combine the water, 1 cup soy sauce, cloves, peppercorns, star anise, and maple extract. Bring to a boil. Baste the pork belly all over with the sauce you made in the jar. Place in steamer basket over the boiling liquid in the pot with a tight-fitting lid to cover. Steam 45 minutes, basting occasionally until tender. Transfer the pork belly to a baking sheet. Set your oven to broil. Keeping a close watch and continuing to baste occasionally, brown all sides until it begins to crisp. Remove from the oven and allow to rest 15 to 20 minutes before slicing. Serve nice and hot.

Alaska Style Beans

INGREDIENTS:

- 1 lb. dry pinto beans (Sort carefully and discard sticks, rocks, and beans with skin missing or shriveled, undersized, or discolored. Only keep plump, perfect, flawless beans. Throw away the rest.)
- Enough water to cover by 4 to 5 inches
- 6 c. very rich light stock (chicken, pork, or veal)
- 1 lb. jowl bacon, medium dice
- 1 large sweet onion, small dice
- 2 medium carrots, small dice
- 4 ribs celery, small dice
- 8 cloves of garlic, coarsely chopped
- 2 bay leaves
- 1 tbsp. cumin seeds, toasted and ground fresh
- 1 tsp. cayenne pepper
- 1 small sprig fresh thyme
- salt & freshly ground pepper to taste

DIRECTIONS:

Bring the beans to a boil in water in a large pot. Boil for 20 minutes, then turn off the heat. Allow the beans to soak undisturbed for 1 hour and 30 minutes. Drain and rinse thoroughly. In the large pot while the beans drain, add vegetables and jowl bacon. Cook over medium-low heat until sweated and just turning color. Add beans, spices, and herbs to the pot with the stock. Bring to a boil and then reduce heat to a slow, steady simmer. Cook for an hour and then test 3 beans. If they are tender, they are done. Sometimes it will take an extra 20 to 30 minutes. When the beans are tender, adjust seasoning with salt and pepper. Remove bay leaves and any stems left from the fresh thyme, and serve.

Moose Curry

INGREDIENTS:

- 2 lbs. moose meat, cut into 3-inch pieces
- salt & pepper
- 1 c. all-purpose unbleached flour
- ¼ c. mustard oil
- 1 large onion, medium dice
- 6 Roma-style tomatoes, medium dice
- 8 cloves fresh garlic, peeled
- 3 carrots cut in 2-inch rounds
- 1 tbsp. coriander seeds
- 1 tsp. brown mustard seeds
- ½ tsp. black peppercorns
- ½ whole real cinnamon stick
- ½ tsp. whole cardamom pods
- 1 tsp. fenugreek seeds
- ½ tsp. cayenne pepper
- 1½ tbsp. ground turmeric
- 2 tsp. ground ginger
- 2 bay leaves
- tomato paste
- moose stock (beef stock can be substituted)
- 2 c. coconut milk

DIRECTIONS:

In a small pan, combine the coriander, mustard seeds, peppercorns, cinnamon stick (crushed), cardamom, and fenugreek seeds. On medium-low heat, roast the seeds while stirring to keep from browning too fast. Soon as the spices become very fragrant and start to pop and move around, remove from the heat. Allow the spices to cool slightly in the pan. In a spice grinder (or coffee bean grinder), pulse until a powder. Mix in the cayenne pepper, turmeric, and ginger. Set your freshly made curry powder aside, ready to use.

Season the moose meat generously with salt & pepper. Dredge lightly with flour. In a big Dutch oven, brown in the mustard oil just until the flour is golden. Remove to a bowl (add more oil if needed). Stir the curry powder into the oil in the pan. Sauté until it becomes very fragrant. Add in tomato paste and continue to stir and cook until it starts to change color. Be careful not to scorch, by stirring constantly. Add in vegetables, stock, moose meat, and coconut milk along with the bay leaves; stir so everything is evenly distributed in the pot. Put on the lid and bake in a 325-degree oven for 1 hour. Remove pot from the oven and test the vegetables and meat for tenderness. Salt & pepper to taste.

DESSERTS

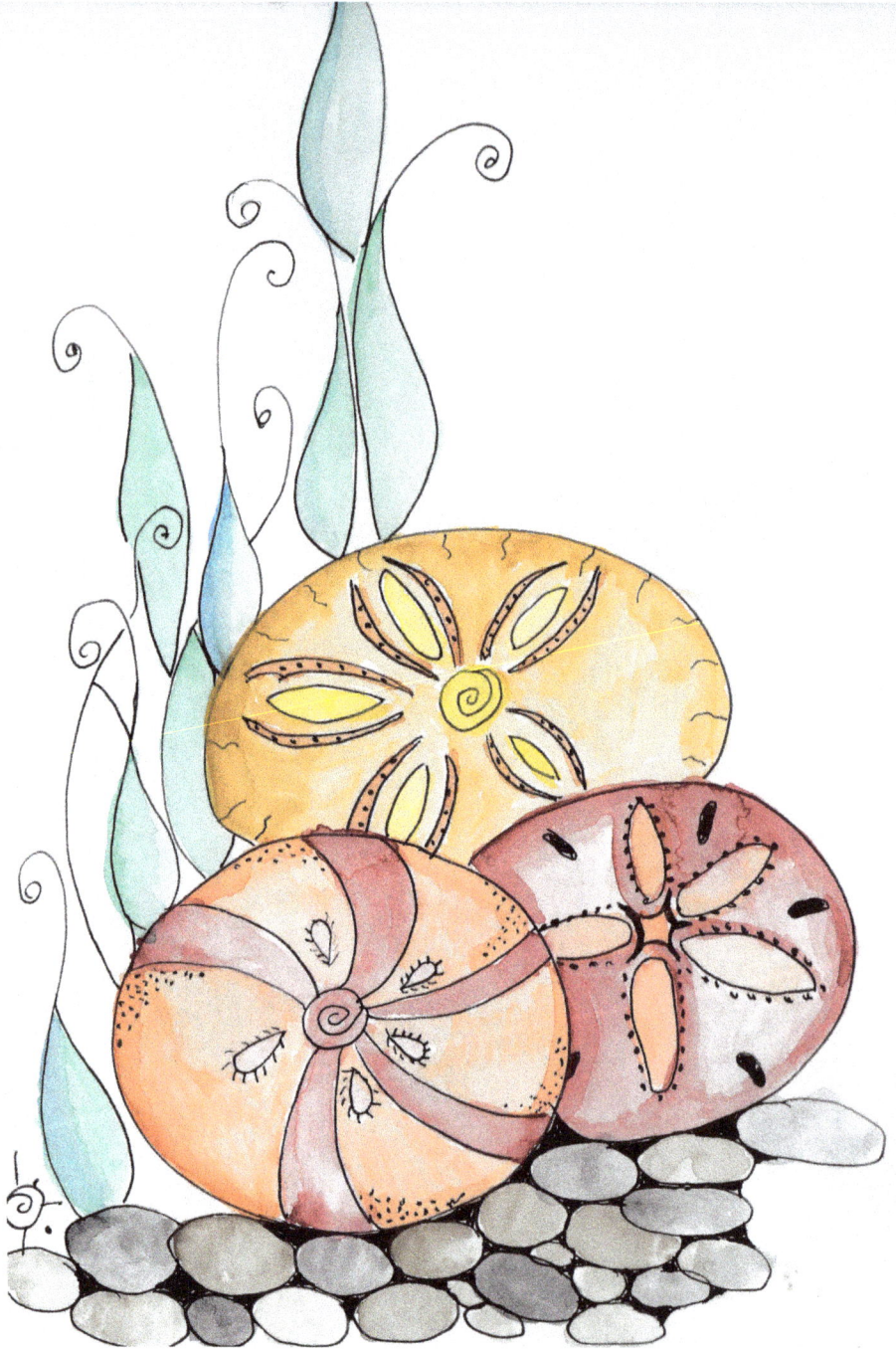

Fresh Pumpkin Pie & Crust Recipe

INGREDIENTS:

- 2 c. mashed, roasted pumpkin
- ¼ c. softened butter
- 12 oz. heavy cream
- 2 eggs, beaten
- ¾ c. packed brown sugar
- 2 tsp. Jamaican allspice
- 2⅔ cups graham flour or unbleached all-purpose flour
- 2 tbsp. brown sugar
- 1 tsp. salt
- 1 c. chilled, unsalted butter
- ½ c. cold water

DIRECTIONS:

Preheat oven to 400 degrees.

Halve pumpkin and scoop out seeds and stringy portions. Cut pumpkin into chunks. In a roasting pan, toss pumpkin chunks with oil and roast 30 to 45 minutes or until tender. Let cool and peel.

In a large bowl, with a hand mixer (or a food processor works well on this, if you have one) mix the pumpkin, allspice, butter, and sugar until smooth." Add one egg at a time and mix until completely incorporated into the pumpkin mixture. Slowly add the cream and mix until combined. Pour into the piecrusts and bake 40 minutes or until knife inserted in the middle comes out clean.

TO MAKE PIECRUSTS: Mix together the flour, sugar, and salt. Cut butter into flour by using a pastry cutter, or a food processor works well as long as you pulse it so the butter doesn't warm up and bind to the flour. Add 1 tablespoon of water at a time to the mixture. Mix dough and repeat until dough is moist enough to hold together.

Divide dough in half and, with lightly floured hands, shape into two balls. Place a ball of dough on a sheet of lightly floured plastic wrap and sprinkle the top of the dough lightly with flour. Place another sheet of plastic wrap on top of the ball of dough and roll out dough to ⅛-inch thickness. Remove the top sheet of plastic wrap from the dough. Use the bottom sheet to transfer the crust to a 9-inch pie pan, turning the dough upside-down so that the plastic wrap is on the top, and then remove it. Lightly press the dough evenly into the pie pan. With a sharp knife, trim off any of the excess dough hanging off around the edge of the pie pan. You can use a fork to press around the outer edge of the dough to make a decorative outer crust. Makes 2 pies.

Wenches' Lemon Meringue Pie
with Shortbread Cookie Crust

INGREDIENTS:

- lemon zest of 3 lemons
- juice of 3 lemons, or ½ c.
- 4 egg yolks (reserve whites for meringue)
- ⅓ c. cornstarch
- 1½ c. water
- 1⅓ c. sugar
- 1 tsp. pure vanilla extract
- ¼ teaspoon salt
- 3 tbsp. butter

DIRECTIONS:

In a medium saucepan, combine cornstarch, water, sugar, egg yolks, and salt. Whisk to combine. Turn heat on medium and, stirring constantly, bring mixture to a boil. Boil for 1 minute or until thickened; take care not to let it scorch. Remove from heat and gently stir in butter, lemon juice, vanilla, and zest until well combined; return to heat and cook a little longer until it is once again thick. Pour mixture into pie shell and top with meringue while filling is still hot. Make sure meringue completely covers filling and that it goes right up to the edge of the crust. Bake for 10 to 12 minutes or until meringue is golden. Remove from oven and cool on a wire rack. Make sure pie is cooled completely before slicing.

Meringue Topping

INGREDIENTS:

- 4 egg whites
- 1 pinch cream of tartar
- 2 tbsp. raw sugar

DIRECTIONS:

Place egg whites and cream of tartar in the bowl of a stand mixer fitted with the whisk attachment, or in a bowl with hand mixer or wire whisk. Beat egg whites until soft peaks form and then gradually add sugar and continue beating until stiff peaks form, approximately 1 to 2 minutes. Use to top lemon filling.

Cookie piecrust

INGREDIENTS:

- 2 c. shortbread cookie crumbs
- ¼ c. melted butter
- ¼ c. raw sugar

DIRECTIONS:

In a mixing bowl, combine ingredients, then press firmly into a 9-inch pie pan and bake for 10 to 15 minutes in a 350-degree oven to set crust.

Sweet Potato Fried Pies
and Alaskan Birch Syrup Whipped Cream,
Garnished with Peanut Brittle Dust

INGREDIENTS:

CRUST:

- 2 c. all-purpose unbleached flour
- ⅔ c. chilled lard
- 1 tsp. salt
- 6 tbsp. cold water
- flour water (water & flour combined to make a thin paste)

FILLING:

- 2 c. cooked and mashed sweet potato
- ½ c. brown sugar
- 1 tbsp. Jamaican allspice
- 2 tbsp. butter, room temperature (soft)

WHIPPED CREAM:

- 1 pint heavy whipping cream
- ¼ c. Alaskan birch syrup

DIRECTIONS:

TO MAKE CRUST: Combine flour and salt. Cut in chilled lard until combined with flour, working quickly so the fat does not warm up and combine with the flour, which makes your crust tough. Add chilled water and combine to make a ball. Wrap in plastic and let rest in the fridge until ready to roll out into about 5-inch circles about ⅛-inch thick.

TO MAKE FILLING: Combine all ingredients completely in a medium-size bowl.

TO MAKE PIES: Place a generous tablespoon of filling on one half of the 5-inch crusts. Moisten around the edge of the crust with flour water. Fold crust in half over the filling and pinch along the edges to seal. Place pies on a baking sheet to let seals around the pies dry a little, about 30 minutes, to keep your filling inside while frying. Fry in $1/2$ inch of oil on medium heat, being careful to not get it too hot as to burn your crust and not warm the insides, and being sure not to have heat too low or your pies will soak up oil and become greasy. When pies are brown, remove to paper towel or wire rack. Serve with whipped cream flavored with Alaskan birch syrup and dusted with ground peanut brittle.

TO MAKE WHIPPED CREAM: Chill bowl and mixer beaters in the fridge until cold. Pour heavy cream and birch syrup into chilled bowl and beat with a hand mixer on high speed until stiff peaks are formed, approximately 8 to 12 minutes.

WENCHY HALLOWEEN TREATS
(POPCORN BALLS & CARAMEL APPLES)

INGREDIENTS:
POPCORN BALLS:

- 1 c. raw cane sugar
- ¼ c. pure Alaskan Birch Syrup
- ¼ c. water
- 1 tsp. salt
- 1 tbsp. butter
- 2 qt. popped popcorn
- butter, for hands and pan

CARAMEL APPLES:

- 1 c. finely chopped salted peanuts
- ½ c. butter
- 2 c. firmly packed dark brown sugar
- 1 c. maple syrup
- dash salt
- 1½ c. heavy cream
- 1 tsp. pure vanilla
- 10 apples, washed, dried
- 10 Popsicle sticks

DIRECTIONS:
POPCORN BALLS:

In a 2-quart saucepan, combine sugar, birch syrup, water, salt, and butter. Cook to the hard ball stage (about 250 degrees on candy thermometer), stirring occasionally. Remove from heat. Working quickly, stir in popped corn and turn into a buttered pan. With buttered hands, shape into balls and place on waxed paper to cool.

Makes about 6 popcorn balls.

CARAMEL APPLES:
Place peanuts in small bowl. Set aside.

Melt butter in 2-quart saucepan; add brown sugar, maple syrup, and salt. Cook over medium heat, stirring occasionally, until mixture comes to a full boil (10 to 12 minutes). Stir in heavy cream. Continue cooking, stirring occasionally, until small amount of mixture dropped into ice water forms a firm ball, or candy thermometer reaches 245 degrees (20 to 25 minutes). Remove from heat; stir in vanilla.

Insert stick into the stem side of the apple through the core; dip apples into caramel mixture. Dip one end of each apple into peanuts. Place onto buttered waxed paper.

FRUIT STEW WITH SWEET VANILLA DUMPLINGS

INGREDIENTS:

FRUIT STEW:

- 1 c. prunes, 1 c. dried apricots, 1 c. dried apples, 1 c. dried cherries, 1 c. dried currants, 1 c. golden raisins
- 2 tbsp. butter
- 3 vanilla beans
- 3 cinnamon sticks
- 2 c. spiced rum
- 4 c. cider

DUMPLINGS:

- 1 c. unbleached all-purpose flour
- 1 c. cake flour
- 2 tbsp. raw cane sugar
- vanilla beans (from the stew, scrape the seeds from the inside out)
- 1 tsp. baking powder
- ½ tsp. salt
- ¾ c. cream

DIRECTIONS:

TO MAKE STEW: Combine all ingredients in a large heavy kettle over high heat. Reduce heat to a slow simmer. Cook slowly 1½ to 2 hours, stirring occasionally and adding more cider if it starts to go dry. Remove cinnamon sticks and vanilla beans, scraping the inside out and reserving for the dumplings.

TO MAKE DUMPLINGS: Combine all the dry ingredients in a bowl, cut butter into dry ingredients, add enough cream to make a soft sticky dough. Drop by heaping tablespoons into the simmering fruit stew. Cook on top of the stove covered for 25 minutes, just under a simmer until cooked through.

FIREWEED JELLY CHEESECAKE
WITH LADYFINGER CRUST

INGREDIENTS:

- 1 lb. mascarpone cheese
- 1 lb. sour cream
- $\frac{1}{4}$ c. butter
- 4 eggs
- $\frac{1}{4}$ c. fireweed jelly
- $\frac{1}{2}$ c. raw cane sugar
- $3\frac{1}{2}$ c. coarsely ground ladyfingers
- $\frac{1}{4}$ c. melted butter
- $\frac{1}{4}$ c. sugar
- 1 c. fireweed jelly

DIRECTIONS:

Combine in a bowl the ladyfingers, melted butter, and sugar for the crust. Press crust mixture firmly into a 9-inch springform pan evenly. Bake crust 15 minutes in a 350-degree oven and let cool on a wire rack. In a large bowl with an electric mixer or in a stand mixer, whip the mascarpone, sour cream, butter, and cane sugar until light and fluffy. While continuing to mix on medium speed, add one egg at a time; after eggs are combined, add the jelly and continue mixing until it is incorporated. Pour batter into springform pan over the crust and bake in 350-degree oven for 45 minutes, or until knife inserted comes out clean. Let cool completely, then cover top with the jelly and let set for 1 hour. Slice and serve garnished with fireweed flowers.

Apricot White Chocolate Chip
with Pecan Cookies

INGREDIENTS:

- 4½ c. all-purpose unbleached flour
- 2 tsp. baking soda
- 2 tsp. butter flavor popcorn salt
- 2 c. soft butter
- 1½ c. raw sugar
- 1½ c. firmly packed brown sugar
- 2 tbsp. black rum
- 4 duck eggs
- 4 c. of the best quality white chocolate chips
- 2 c. pecans, quartered and toasted, then cooled
- 2 c. dried apricots, quartered

DIRECTIONS:

Sift together the baking soda, salt, and flour in a bowl and reserve. In a stand mixer, whip the sugars and rum with the butter until light and fluffy on a higher speed. Add the eggs one at a time to the butter mixture and incorporate it completely before adding the next egg. Once the egg and butter mixture are very light and fluffy, add all the other ingredients to the stand mixer. Mix on low speed until all the nuts, apricots, and chocolate chips are evenly distributed in the dough. Let the dough rest 30 minutes. Line baking sheets with parchment paper and preheat the oven to 375 degrees. With a tablespoon scoop or measuring spoon, place balls of cookie dough on the cookie sheet. Leave enough room between because it does spread a little as it bakes. Bake 11 minutes if you want them soft in the middle, 14 minutes for perfect golden brown (depending on oven). Let sit 3 to 5 minutes on baking sheet and then remove to cooling racks.

Rum & Chocolate Eclairs

INGREDIENTS:

- 1 c. butter
- 2 c. water
- 1 tsp. raw sugar
- 2 c. unbleached all-purpose flour
- ½ tsp. popcorn salt
- 4 duck eggs, room temperature
- 4½ c. whole milk
- 2 vanilla beans, scraped
- ¼ c. Lyle's golden syrup
- ⅓ c. cornstarch
- 1 c. heavy whipping cream
- ½ c. raw sugar
- 1 c. good quality semisweet or dark chocolate
- ¼ c. butter
- ¼ c. black rum
- ¼ c. water
- 2 c. confectioner's sugar
- edible gold leaf

DIRECTIONS:

Start first with the filling by whisking the milk into the cornstarch slowly so there are no lumps. Add the golden syrup and the seeds from inside 2 vanilla pods to the milk in a pot, and keep whisking as you heat on medium high until thick like pudding (reuse the pods in a jar of sugar to make vanilla sugar). Strain the filling through a sieve to remove any lumps. Chill completely.

In a stand mixer or by hand mixer, whip the heavy cream until foamy and starting to thicken. Add the ½ cup raw sugar and continue to beat until stiff peaks form. Fold whipped cream into the chilled pudding mixture, being careful to mix evenly without losing the air out of it. Fill pastry bags with the filling, fitted with a filling tip. Chill in the refrigerator until ready to fill the eclairs (this can be done the night before).

Next make the pate a choux dough by bringing the water, 1 cup butter, 1 tsp. raw sugar, and popcorn salt to a boil. Whisk in the flour so there are no lumps. Switch to a wooden spoon or heat-proof spatula and continue stirring and cooking the flour mixture until it comes together as a glossy dough. Remove from heat. Place dough into a stand mixer, and on medium speed beat in the duck eggs one at a time until it becomes a loose, very thick dough. Fill pastry bags fitted with a large star tip with the dough. Pipe the dough in 3-inch strips on a parchment-lined baking sheet. Place the pans in a 450-degree oven for 15 minutes, then turn the oven down to 325 degrees and bake another 20 minutes until golden brown and dry inside. Remove to cooling racks and allow to cool completely before filling (this can be done the night before).

Next, make the chocolate glaze by bringing the ¼ cup butter and ¼ cup water to a boil and removing from heat. Add in the chocolate and stir until smooth. Whisk in the confectioner's sugar and rum. Stir until very smooth and no lumps.

To assemble the éclairs, poke a hole in one end of the éclair with the filling tip and fill; do the same on the other end of the éclair. Make sure filling reaches the middle of the éclair. Repeat with the rest of the éclairs. Dip the top of each éclair in the warm chocolate icing. Decorate the top of the chocolate with a touch of gold and serve.

Galley Wench Style Tiramisu

INGREDIENTS:

- 3 duck egg whites
- 6 duck egg yolks
- ¼ c. raw sugar, plus 2 tbsp.
- 1 c. heavy whipping cream
- ¼ c. Lyle's golden syrup
- ½ tsp. salt
- 8 oz. mascarpone cheese at room temperature
- 1 c. freshly pulled espresso, cooled to room temperature
- 2 tbsp. black spiced rum
- 3-4 dozen ladyfingers, store-bought or homemade
- 1 c. grated dark chocolate or shavings

DIRECTIONS:

Separate 6 eggs, and place 3 of the egg whites in the bowl of a stand mixer, and 6 egg yolks in another. Beat the egg whites until they become foamy and begin to turn white. Add in the sugar and continue to beat until just the beginning of stiff peaks are forming. Set aside in another bowl. In the stand mixer bowl, stir in the heavy whipped cream with the golden syrup and salt until dissolved. Whip the cream mixture until it becomes a stiff whipped cream (be careful not to overwhip and make butter). Set the whipped cream aside in another bowl. In the same stand mixer bowl, whip the egg yolks until they become light in color and very fluffy. Whisk in the mascarpone cheese until very light and airy. Next, carefully fold in first the whipped cream and last the whipped egg whites until evenly combined, while being very careful not to deflate. Time to assemble: In a bowl, mix together the rum and the fresh espresso. Give each ladyfinger a quick dunk in the coffee and then lay them together to cover the bottom of a flat 8-inch x 8-inch-square dish. Cover the layer of ladyfingers with half the mascarpone mixture and spread evenly. Cover the mascarpone layer with another layer of dunked ladyfingers. Next, add the rest of the mascarpone mixture and spread evenly. Chill one hour to overnight. Sprinkle the top with the grated chocolate. Cut and serve.

Taro Cake

INGREDIENTS:

- ½ c. raw sugar
- 1 c. brown sugar
- ½ c. grapeseed oil
- 2 duck eggs
- 1¾ c. sifted, unbleached, all-purpose flour
- 1 tsp. baking soda
- 2 tsp. Jamaican allspice
- ¼ tsp. popcorn salt
- ⅓ c. whole milk
- 1 c. cooked and mashed roasted taro
- purple food color
- ½ c. chopped macadamia nuts
- 1½ c. confectioner's sugar
- 3 tbsp. coconut cream

DIRECTIONS:

Bake the taro with skin on in a 420-degree oven, 45 minutes to 1½ hours, until a fork inserts easily to the middle. Allow to cool, then scoop the soft fluffy taro out of the skin with a spoon. Sift together the flour, baking soda, salt, and allspice. In a stand mixer, whip the taro with the oil and sugar until the sugar is dissolved into the potatoes. Whip in one egg at a time to make a fluffy mixture. Add in flour and milk and continue to mix until you have a nice batter. (But don't overmix or it will make a tough cake.) Bake at 350 degrees in two buttered loaf pans for 1 hour. After baking, remove from loaf pans and cool on a wire rack until room temperature. Mix the confectioner's sugar and coconut cream to make a glaze. Drizzle glaze over the loaves and sprinkle with the chopped macadamia nuts.

Galley Wench Style Flan

INGREDIENTS:

- 1 c. raw sugar
- 4 duck eggs
- 1 (14 ounce) can sweetened condensed milk
- 1 (12 fluid ounce) can evaporated milk
- 1 c. heavy whipping cream
- 1 tbsp. black rum

DIRECTIONS:

In a medium saucepan over medium-low heat, melt sugar until liquefied and golden in color. Carefully pour hot syrup into a 9-inch round glass baking dish, turning the dish to evenly coat the bottom and sides. Set aside.

In a large bowl, beat eggs. Beat in condensed milk, evaporated milk, cream, and rum until smooth. Pour egg mixture into baking dish. Place the baking dish in a large enough roasting dish to fill halfway up the side with water.

Bake in preheated oven, 350 degrees for 60 minutes. Let cool completely.

To serve, carefully invert on serving plate with edges, once completely cool.

The Galley Wench's Basic White Bread

INGREDIENTS:

- 4 c. unbleached all-purpose flour
- 1 pkg. active dry yeast or 2½ tbsp.
- 2 tbsp. raw cane sugar or brown sugar
- 2 tsp. salt
- 2 tbsp. melted butter or olive oil
- 1½ c. warm water
- extra flour for hands and kneading surface

DIRECTIONS:

Combine all the ingredients in a large mixing bowl, and with your hands mix it well until all the flour is combined with the liquids. Sprinkle your kneading surface lightly with flour and turn out your dough onto it. Dust the top of the dough lightly with flour. To begin kneading, grasp the edge of the dough opposite the side that is closest to you, and pull it up; fold it in half, pressing down and pushing forward with your hands made into fists. Turn the dough one-quarter turn and do the same; if dough begins to stick to kneading surface or your hands, dust lightly with additional flour. Continue this method of kneading for approximately 10 minutes until dough is smooth and elastic. In a lightly oiled bowl, place dough and roll it over so that top and bottom are oiled. Place a piece of plastic wrap or a clean dish towel loosely over the bowl and let rise in a warm place for 1 to 1½ hours, or until doubled in size. Punch down the dough to deflate. Knead once again but for about 5 minutes. Cut dough in half and place one half on kneading surface; shape it with your hands to form a loaf and place in a greased loaf pan. Repeat with other half of the dough and return loaves to warm place to rise once more. Bake 45 minutes in a 350-degree oven. Remove from oven and pan to a cooling rack. Let cool before you slice it, because if it is hot it is still cooking, even after being removed from the oven. Recipe makes 2 loaves.

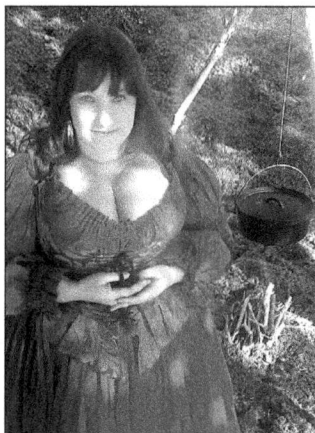

Ony Worel

Born in Washington state in 1972, Ony spent her childhood as an apprentice in father Theodore W. Worel's restaurant kitchen. She arrived on the Kenai Peninsula at the age of 14 and obtained her first job cooking and caring for the little girl of a family of setnet commercial fishermen. This placement started her career in studying, learning, and developing Alaska Galley Wench Style cuisine. For 30 years, Ony has studied local ingredients and classic techniques of cooking and has worked in restaurants, lodges, fish camps, and hunting camps. She has also taught cooking over her live radio show, The Galley Wench's Cooking Show, and through local community schools.

www.ingramcontent.com/pod-product-compliance
Lightning Source LLC
Chambersburg PA
CBHW071854090426
42811CB00004B/597